Life Beyond
100

Also by C. Norman Shealy, M.D., Ph.D.

90 Days to Stress-Free Living: A Day-by-Day Health Plan, Including Exercises, Diet, and Relaxation Techniques

The Creation of Health: The Emotional, Psychological, and Spiritual Responses That Promote Health and Healing
(with Caroline Myss)

Sacred Healing: The Curing Power of Energy and Spirituality

The Illustrated Encyclopedia of Healing Remedies

Life Beyond

100

Secrets of the Fountain of Youth

C. NORMAN SHEALY, M.D., Ph.D.

Jeremy P. Tarcher/Penguin

a member of Penguin Group (USA) Inc.

New York

JEREMY P. TARCHER / PENGUIN
Published by the Penguin Group
Penguin Group (USA) Inc., 375 Hudson Street, New York, New York 10014, USA •
Penguin Group (Canada), 90 Eglinton Avenue East, Suite 700, Toronto, Ontario M4P 2Y3,
Canada (a division of Pearson Penguin Canada Inc.) • Penguin Books Ltd, 80 Strand,
London WC2R 0RL, England • Penguin Ireland, 25 St Stephen's Green, Dublin 2, Ireland
(a division of Penguin Books Ltd) • Penguin Group (Australia), 250 Camberwell Road,
Camberwell, Victoria 3124, Australia (a division of Pearson Australia Group Pty Ltd) •
Penguin Books India Pvt Ltd, 11 Community Centre, Panchsheel Park, New Delhi–110 017, India •
Penguin Group (NZ), Cnr Airborne and Rosedale Roads, Albany, Auckland 1310, New Zealand
(a division of Pearson New Zealand Ltd) • Penguin Books (South Africa) (Pty) Ltd,
24 Sturdee Avenue, Rosebank, Johannesburg 2196, South Africa

Penguin Books Ltd, Registered Offices: 80 Strand, London WC2R 0RL, England

First trade paperback edition 2006
Copyright © 2005 by C. Norman Shealy, M.D., Ph.D.
Foreword © 2005 by Caroline Myss

The Library of Congress catalogued the hardcover edition as follows:

Life beyond 100 : secrets of the fountain of youth / C. Norman Shealy.
p.   cm.
Includes bibliographical references and index.
ISBN 1-58542-431-5
1. Longevity   2. Health.   I. Title: Life beyond one hundred.   II. Title.
RA776.75.S458   2005   2005054941
613.2—dc22

ISBN 1-58542-523-0 (paperback edition)
Printed in the United States of America
1   3   5   7   9   10   8   6   4   2

Book design by Meighan Cavanaugh

Most Tarcher/Penguin books are available at special quantity discounts for bulk purchase for sales promotions, premiums, fund-raising, and educational needs. Special books or book excerpts also can be created to fit specific needs. For details, write Penguin Group (USA) Inc. Special Markets, 375 Hudson Street, New York, NY 10014.

While the author has made every effort to provide accurate telephone numbers and Internet addresses at the time of publication, neither the publisher nor the author assumes any responsibility for errors, or for changes that occur after publication. Further, the publisher does not have any control over and does not assume any responsibility for author or third-party websites or their content.

Neither the publisher nor the author is engaged in rendering professional advice or services to the individual reader. The ideas, procedures, and suggestions contained in this book are not intended as a substitute for consulting with a physician. All matters regarding health require medical supervision. Neither the author nor the publisher shall be liable or responsible for any loss or damage allegedly arising from any information or suggestion in this book.

CONTENTS

FOREWORD:
YOUTHFUL AGING

Caroline Myss

Reading *Life Beyond 100: Secrets of the Fountain of Youth* is like entering a secret chamber deep within the human spirit that contains the precious details about who we are and how we function, when it is understood that we are first and foremost beings of energy contained within physical form. Yet, if understood deeply, the revelations about the power Möbius that exists between the human energy and the physical body could indeed extend the experience of physical life well past age 100, perhaps even past age 120, or even—dare your imagination reach this far—age 140.

I would fully expect a person's reaction to be "impossible," and up until now, that was not only true—it *was* impossible. But, just because something has always been "true" does not necessarily mean that it is also "truth." Rather, what it suggests is that we had not yet reached one of those rare "open-minded" windows of opportunity in human evolution where a new concept, or scientific discovery, or grand paradigm that challenges the core of reality can slip into the collective unconscious. But we did experience such a window of opportunity during these past forty years that initiated a revolution in thought that reached every domain of our society, including the field of health. From this revolution, the holistic health movement emerged, and immediately, C. Norman Shealy, M.D., Ph.D., became one of its foremost leaders in research and pioneering the field of energy medicine, including medical intuition, which is how we met twenty years ago. By that time, Norm was already established as an authority in the alternative medical community, having authored six books by 1984. Since then, he has authored an additional fifteen. Hence, this is his twenty-second book, and in my opinion, his finest.

The idea of living well past age 100 as a healthy and vital person, as a "youthful centenarian," is radical even for proponents of a healthy lifestyle that is complete with all the proper alternative health-style requirements. The missing ingredient, however, in all previous books on good nutrition, exercise, vitamin intake, and other physical requirements is that they neglected what could be the most essential component of the human being, which is to understand the "eternal ingredient," the nature of the human energy system.

Here is the fundamental truth that Norm examines as a physician, a scientist, and as a contemporary "mystic in the field of medicine": Energy does not age and you are composed of 100 percent energy, as well as matter. Unlike the mathematical equation of how much water you are, and matter and protein and salt, and all the other physical chemicals that form the body, energy is the only "nonsubstance substance" that is equal to the percentage of your body parts *and* does not age. Energy is also a conscious substance— overlapping into the domain of the spirit. As such, this substance, this vital part of your being, requires as much care and attention as your physical body. And in some cases, your energy and spirit require more attention. Simply put, we have arrived at a time in our evolution as a species at which we must now approach who we are and what we are as a species with the understanding that we are primarily systems of energy that must be integrated in a congruent form with the physical body. One need not even hold to a spiritual paradigm for that truth to be respected; spirituality is an add-on, a personal practice that an individual maintains within his or her lifestyle. Understanding the human energy system as the electromagnetic companion to the physical body should be taken for what it is—solid science.

Life Beyond 100 builds upon that truth as a given and introduces the reader to a domain of power—and self-empowerment—that exists as untapped potential that can, once released, slow down the aging process, not as a result of a vitamin or an exercise, but as a result of understanding the functioning mechanism between the physical body and the electromagnetic system, which is composed of emotions, the psyche, and the human spirit. In keeping with his deep regard for science, Norm presents the research of scientists in the field of electromagnetics and other related fields, which shows that other great minds are tackling this frontier of thought. And, in keeping with his ever-present role as a physician, he grounds this material in his commonsense approach to health care, which includes examining basic self-care practices such as nutrition, diet, exercise, sleep patterns, depression monitoring, and vitamin intake.

But in addition to those regulators of health, Norm highlights the critical role that self-esteem plays in governing the quality of one's health, and I chose the word *governing* quite deliberately. For me, drawing upon my own work and research as a medical intuitive, I have concluded that self-esteem is the "make or break" power of the individual. Self-esteem is the interior substance that connects the psyche to the spirit, if one can even suggest that there is a bridge of connection between the psyche and the spirit. If such a bridge could be imagined just for the sake of discussion, then it is a person's sense of self that provides that individual with the courage he or she needs to unleash the power of his or her spirit. It is that specific power—unleashed and unlimited—that Norm is referring to in this brilliant and groundbreaking book when he describes exercises such as the Rings of Fire, Air, Earth, Water, and Crystal that he discovered over a decade ago. The Rings engage a field of contact between the subtle energy currents of one's more potent energy field and one's physical body. These are the circuits that hold the potential to influence the "speed" at which illnesses ordinarily heal—emphasis on the word *speed*. Speed can be influenced, as proponents of energy medicine and positive imagery already believe. They have yet to learn, however, as they will in this text, how powerful that practice is once a map of energetic data is applied to energetic visualization, connecting the power of the mind to the density of the body with an exercise in energy medicine. The Ring of Crystal, for example, activates an etheric field of subtle currents of energy that significantly reduces chemical free radicals, which are major contributors to "aging." Each of these unique rings has specific youth-enhancing energetics.

As I gathered my thoughts and notes in preparation to writing the foreword to *Life Beyond 100*, I ended up with a much-too-long list of topics I wanted to include because I realized how groundbreaking and significant they are in this world. I felt like adding a paragraph, or three or ten, with arrows pointing to certain pages, highlighting the importance of what Norm has revealed to the world in this book, much of which should rightly be noted as "scientific revelation." I especially wanted to do that because I understand—and that isn't even big enough—I know at a soul level that what Norm is saying is *truth* opposed to true or possible or maybe. I know in part from my own background in medical intuition, but also because of how I have come to understand the nature and workings of the human spirit. I know that the human spirit is a living force that is ageless and that the body takes its commands from the authority, strength, and health of the spirit. Obviously there isn't a book on health in the world that can outrun the will of God if our time has come, so to speak. But what if we have the choice to live equal to the quality of care we pour into ourselves? After all, our body, mind, spirit, and energy system are as much a classroom of learning as are the lessons provided by the world around us. That choice may well exist now, but until now—until we were ready to ascend to our next level of understanding *and* conduct ourselves as conscious energy systems—that quality of choice could not have been animated because, quite simply, we lacked the wherewithal to manage it.

Norm's premise that we can live far longer than current science suggests does bring up the question of whether or not we *want* to live that long. That's another issue entirely and quite a personal one. Obviously, only you can decide that. Still, in the process of pondering that question, *if* you truly ponder that question to its fullest extent, you will come to terms with the fact that you *do* have choice in terms of how long and how well you want to live. You'll know this because the thought of living well past 100 years might terrify you, and if so, that fear indicates the possibility that you *could* if you wanted to. Or you might find yourself elated at the possibility that you could extend your life another—well, who knows how many years, depending upon how old you are when you are reading this. And that choice is pure power.

I've said this before, and no doubt I will say it many, many more times in the years to come: I consider Norm Shealy to be one of the geniuses of our era. *Life Beyond 100* is a masterpiece because not only does Norm include the human spirit in his paradigm of health; he also describes a full and complete health program *for* the human spirit as well as the human body. And as is typical of the work of this wizard-genius-scientist-mystic-physician, he is once again leading the health community to its next plateau of research in the field of health and human consciousness.

CAROLINE MYSS,
author of *Anatomy of the Spirit, Sacred Contracts,*
and *Invisible Acts of Power*

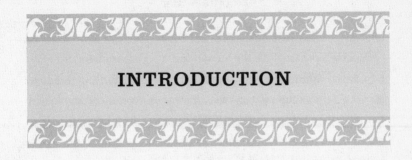

INTRODUCTION

HOW LONG DO YOU WANT TO LIVE?

The search for youth and eternal life is perhaps as old as civilization: Ponce de León's explorations to locate the Fountain of Youth, the quest for the Holy Grail, the alchemist's attempt to convert lead into gold, and most especially, the search for the Philosopher's Stone are all variations of a grand search for the secret of life. It is interesting that as people pursued this mystery, evolving alchemists became scientists; out of their work came chemistry, metallurgy, and pharmacology. For several hundred years these sciences have dominated the Western world. But in the past decade, even some medical scientists have turned to anti-aging research and others to spiritual revitalization. Suppose there is a mysterious path to health and longer life? A true Fountain of Youth?

One of Sigmund Freud's most accurate and startling discoveries about the human psyche was the pervasiveness of the "death wish." Dr. Eric Berne took this idea further with his concept that we determine the circumstances of our death—at what age and by what cause—early in our lives. For more than ten years before his death, Berne told colleagues that his life contract called for him to die at the age of sixty of a heart attack. And he did just that! Elvis Presley apparently believed that he would die at age forty-two, the age at which his mother died. His expectation was fulfilled.

In having worked with more than thirty thousand chronically ill patients, I have observed depression and poor self-esteem to be at the root of most problems. Clinically, we know that at least 40 percent of Americans are depressed enough to need therapy; I now suspect that another 40 percent are at least depressed enough that Freud's idea of a death wish is alive and well.

While this book may not appeal to those with few emotional reserves, or to those who have set a life contract to die early, I believe that significant numbers of energetic, enthusiastic individuals are ready to redefine old age, providing a new concept of longevity. These may live healthily to a minimum of 100 years, some to 120. And if they embrace the essential activities encouraged by my research, they may live healthily 120 to 160 years, just by adding a few simple activities to their daily lives. These individuals may truly set the stage for Homo noeticus, as defined by Caroline Myss. Essentially Homo noeticus will be the next evolutionary stage after Homo sapiens, adding intuition as an active sixth sense. They will not consider themselves "elderly" until at least 120 years of age.

. . .

THERE ARE SEVERAL "GAMES" AND TESTS OF LONGEVITY to be found on the Internet, some by insurance companies. According to one of these tests, my life expectancy is 100, while another gives me 116 years: an estimate that comes close to my belief about the potential for human longevity. Consider the current average life expectancy in the United States: 76.9 years. Now consider that you may increase your life expectancy in the following ways:

THE LIFE-EXTENSION CHART*

Average life expectancy	76.9 years
Add to Average Life Expectancy, in years:	
Being a woman	2.6
Not smoking	6.0
Body Mass Index between 19 and 24	6.0
No street drugs	1.5
Average alcohol intake of one drink per day	3.0
Exercise at least 7 hours per week	6.0
Average life expectancy for a woman	101.0
Average life expectancy for a man	98.4

(If you are a married man, add 2.6 additional years for a total of 101 years. Marriage does not help women live longer!)

*The statistics for current longevity are based on information from National Center for Health Statistics, *Health, United States, 1993* (Hyattsville, MD).

These simple commonsense habits give you a potential of living well to 101 years.

Now, how do you add another 39 years?

THE FOLLOWING THREE SUGGESTIONS AND THEIR ASSO-ciated benefits to longevity are reasonable expectations based on my extensive review of literature related to **DHEA, calcitonin, and free radicals.*** These will be discussed in later chapters, but for now, DHEA can be defined as the most critical hormone for evaluating your stress reserves. Calcitonin is the hormone essential for maintaining your skeleton, to avoid osteoporosis, a common cause of death in the elderly. (Over 90 percent of individuals "burn out" slowly after age thirty, so that by age eighty most individuals are totally depleted.) Free radicals, ultimately part of all disease and aging, are the metabolic chemicals that oxidize the body.

The three rules for increasing longevity are:

Keep your DHEA level healthy	add 13 years
Keep your calcitonin level optimal	add 13 years
Keep your free radicals low	add 13 years
Average life expectancy	140 years

There is, of course, a genetic component to one's life expectancy, which may add or subtract about twenty years. Thus, all health-conscious individuals should live at least 120 years, while

---

*Bold-faced terms in the text appear in the Glossary.

those with the best genetic potential could live to be 160! Sound crazy? Not to everyone. In November 2003, *Discover* magazine ran an article featuring gerontologist Steve Austad of the University of Idaho, who believes that a 150-year life span is quite feasible. Perhaps future discoveries will extend this potential even further. But for now, the evidence I will present in this book supports the 140-year average potential.

HOW I ARRIVED AT THE ESSENCE OF THIS BOOK

In 1972, I had just completed my first year of transition from neurosurgeon to "comprehensive" physician, expanding my ideas of electrical therapy for pain control into the realms of behavioral modification, stress reduction, biofeedback, and self-care. These were somewhat revolutionary concepts then.

In the fall of that same year, I attended my first ARE® (Association for Research and Enlightenment) Conference, "A Week of Attunement," at Virginia Beach, Virginia. To a great extent, that week was, for me, the beginning of the "rupture of the mental hymen" as described by Andrija Puharic. I became acquainted with the work of Edgar Cayce, castor-oil packs, color therapy, past-life therapy, and many more classic Cayce approaches to health. I had my first out-of-body experience during a harp concert by Joel Andrews and a prolonged cosmic intuitive "knowing" after a past-life-therapy session with Dr. Lindsey Jacobs. The Cayce concept of "mind as the builder" fit perfectly with my recently acquired philosophy from Ambrose Worrall, "Every thought is a prayer."

In the thirty-plus years that have passed since that conference,

I have had the pleasure of attending ARE® events dozens of times, always leaving feeling enlightened, always feeling "at home" with those at the ARE®. And in fact, it was at a subsequent ARE® workshop in 1975 that I first encountered the concept of **holism,** which led me in 1978 to found the American Holistic Medical Association and later both the Holos® Institutes of Health, Inc., and Holos® University Graduate Seminary. Since then, I have continued to seek safe alternatives to drugs and surgery for the 85 percent of individuals who I believe do not need those approaches.

MY WORK IN ELECTRICAL THERAPY HAS CONTINUED SO that we now know of specific "circuits" in the body for altering the most critical neurochemicals affecting health and longevity. The autonomic nervous system is the "imaginative" nervous system; every cell in the body is replaced within seven years. Cayce describes this process:

To be sure, as it has been indicated again and again, there is that within the physical forces of the body which may be revivified or rejuvenated, if it is kept in a constructive way and manner. This requires, necessarily, the proper thinking, the proper living, the proper application of those influences in the experience of an entity in its associations with everything about a body.[1]

Replacing these cells should lead to constant rejuvenation and increased healthy longevity. And yet Cayce also emphasized the essentials of belief and expectation: "If you have a castor oil personality, take castor oil. If you have a surgical personality, have surgery. You cannot cure a quinine mind of malaria with anything but quinine."[2]

Cayce constantly emphasized that true healing comes from within:

From whence comes the healing? Whether there is administered a drug, a correcting or an adjustment of a subluxation, or the alleviating of a strain upon the muscles, or the revivifying through electrical forces; they are ONE, and the healing comes from WITHIN! Not by the method does the healing come, though the consciousness of the individual IS such that this or that method IS the one that is more effective in the individual case in *arousing the forces from within*. But the METHODS are NOT ideals. The IDEAL must be kept in the proper SOURCE.

Put thy ideal in those things that bespeak of the continuity of life; the regeneration of the spiritual body, the revivifying of the temporal body for SPIRITUAL purposes, that the seed may go forth even as the Teacher gave, "Sin no more, but present thy body as a living sacrifice; holy, acceptable unto Him, for it is a reasonable service."

Hence mind over matter is not to be lightly spoken of, nor is there any disparaging remark to be made as to the ability of the body-physical to be revivified, resuscitated, spiritualized such that there is no reaction that may not be revivified.

Let age only ripen thee. For one is ever as young as the heart and the purpose. Keep sweet. Keep friendly. Keep loving, if ye would keep young.

To be rejuvenated, the body must be kept in a condition of construction; to ever find that the heart, the digestive organs' combination of elimination and assimilation, the hair, the scalp, the nasal, the eye, the ear, the throat, the bronchi, the lungs, the structural forces of the body work as a UNIT, or as ONE! And then we may find, and do find, the body BUILDING, ever.[3]

Cayce also included two subtle electrical devices, the **Radioactive Appliance**—later called the Radial, or Impedance, Device—and the **Wet Cell Battery:** "The use of the Radio-Active Appliance would RE-IONIZE the system, if this is used on evenings before retiring. Not AFTER retiring, but BEFORE retiring; while the body meditates use of the Appliance."[4]

Diet and exercise were also critical elements in the Cayce health program. "At present the diet would be those of the nature carrying the greater rebuilding forces in bloodstream and in nerve tissue. Much then of green vegetable forces, and fish, that are necessary for the body's development. Little of those of starchy or of the heavy forces," Cayce said.[5]

Today holistic practitioners consider attitude, nutrition, exercise, and sleep to be the foundations of health.

Meditation, which has received great attention in the past three decades, was also crucial to Cayce. "Being able to raise *within* the vibrations of individuals to that which is a resuscitating, a revivifying influence and force *through the deep meditation* (the attunement of self to the higher vibrations in Creative Forces), these are manifested in man through the promises that are coming from Creative Forces or Energy itself!"[6]

As we move into the twenty-first century, basic Cayce concepts reinforced by scientific advances of the past sixty years lead me to believe that the "average" American can live healthily for 140 years. Just following the commonsense habits already enumerated should provide an *average* 100 years of life.

I cannot overemphasize the critical necessity of these essentials:

no smoking, Body Mass Index between 19 and 24, optimal nutrition, avoidance of street drugs, moderate alcohol intake, daily physical exercise, and avoidance of elective drugs and medical intervention.

Adding the life-enhancing effects of **human DNA restoration,** to be discussed later, may give you another forty years of active, healthy life. Therein lies the available Fountain of Youth.

While it is quite true that average life expectancy has increased in the past 100 years, it is important that you realize that most of the increase in longevity is related to sanitation and adequate food. Furthermore, the American medical system is now the number-three *cause* of death. I will explore with you the evolution of medical care through excess drug use and the risks to your life and well-being. Then I will help you understand the role of stress and the main chemical effects of excess stress, as well as antidotes to the many stressors we face today. The paradox of nutritional extremes may be of particular interest.

And of course it is important to recognize the prevalence of depression in our society today, with 40 percent of Americans clinically depressed and another 40 percent unhappy. I will offer you a totally safe treatment for depression that is twice as effective as drugs. My work for forty years has emphasized the electrical foundation of life itself and innovative methods for rejuvenating human DNA and the three most important chemicals for a healthy and long life. And there is also a significant story in water as the foundation for life.

Read on as you begin your journey to the Fountain of Youth, a fascinating and fun experience.

Bonne vie!

1

LIFE EXPECTANCY AND
MEDICAL MIRACLES

My great-grandparents were poor southern farmers, fortunate enough to own a small farm. As they aged, they remained active. At 101 years of age, Grandmother Rickard was busy canning in her kitchen. As many farm families did, my great-grandparents managed by turning the farm over to one of their children, in this case, the youngest child, a son, who was responsible for his parents' later years. Indeed, until the societal revolution that began with World War II, most families provided for "old age" this way. It was expected that children would become responsible for aging parents.

In today's society, however, the extended family has become a virtual anomaly. Elderly parents are often rejected or, worse, relegated to "nursing homes" (an oxymoron if I ever saw one). Individuals unfortunate enough to wind up there are often drugged, lonely, depressed. Two different extremes of the nursing-home world were brought to my attention in the early 1970s. One of my colleagues took her social science students to such a "front-end-load" facility in Nevada and performed massage once a week. The death rate at this facility dropped so much within six months that the manager of that living morgue stopped the visits! Meanwhile, in San Francisco, another colleague of mine went to a similar facility and introduced music, dance, and other social activities into the daily lives of residents there. Within six months of her arrival at the nursing home, many of those residents returned home, often living alone!

These two contrasting stories reveal much about the spiritual existential crisis in which we live. People who are happy, active, and engaged in social activities much more often remain happy, active, and healthy, proving that time and age are relative concepts. In fact, to a great extent they are more features of consciousness than they are of physiology. They prompt questions like: Can I afford to get old? and Is it worth getting old if I have great material wealth but no emotional or spiritual vault? Longevity is perhaps a greater spiritual challenge than a physical one.

WE IN THE WESTERN WORLD LIVE IN A PARADOXICAL culture where youth is worshiped and the elderly are often abandoned and warehoused. Medical science emphasizes advances that may enhance life while the media, by and large, have excelled at extolling youth. "Retirement" has been forced on many physically and mentally vibrant leaders at the arbitrary age of sixty-five, while the American Association of Retired Persons (AARP) recruits people beginning at age fifty, "speeding up" the concept of "aged."

As a primarily Judeo-Christian culture, one that, ostensibly, emphasizes the wisdom that comes with advanced years—a culture that celebrates the ages of Methuselah, Jared, and other Biblical greats—we tend toward hypocrisy when the reality of old age intrudes upon our myths. Are the stories of great ages in the Bible pure myth, or is author and Biblical translator Zechariah Sitchen correct in believing that the Elohim/Neflim, who "came down from the sky," actually lived thousands of earth years? Were Methuselah and Jared symbolic or real human beings? Are we intended to live short lives? Did the gods—and in Genesis this additional paradox is emphasized by the seeming polytheism of the phrase "the gods came down"—actually have the secret of eternal life? Did they convey part of their longevity gene to us? And if so, why do we still reject the profound values of aging?

For many decades, the perennial fear of the elderly has been the poverty that seems to be associated with advanced age—another paradox. Overall, those over age sixty-five are, at this time in America, the wealthiest segment of our society. However, those over sixty-five who have not accumulated significant wealth live in states of constant stress, fearing they will outlive their resources.

Overall average life expectancy may have doubled in the past 2,000 years, but life expectancy of those who live to age sixty-five has increased relatively little. People are considered old when they reach age sixty. "He's sixty," someone once said about Paul McCartney. "I have to tell him he shouldn't be looking so good and doing what he's doing."

I ask: What is "old"?

IS MEDICAL CARE RELEVANT?

Dr. Eugene Robin once stated, "The past twenty years have seen an unprecedented accumulation of medical knowledge. This has been accompanied by a growing and unprecedented disillusionment with the application of this knowledge to patient care."[7] Why is this?

For at least the last two thousand years there have been two major philosophical schools of medicine: rationalists and empiricists. The rationalists, or mechanists, have wanted to classify everything into very narrow categories. At the extreme, Galen (a Greek physician in the second century) and others defined each disease as "hot," "cold," "wet," or "dry." Rationalists were often rigid in their thinking, and intolerant of deviation from category. They were, in basic terms, the fundamentalists in society who limited their views, whether in the realms of religion, medicine, science, politics, or economics.

Empiricists, or naturalists (and, at later times, called the eclectics), argued that categories were misleading, that there were infinite possibilities. Empiricists/eclectics tended to be tolerant and broader-minded. Edgar Cayce, for example, represents the ultimate empiricist.

The division between these two schools of thought led to a "battle" that has been thought to be representative of the disagreement between the two schools. This battle was over microorganisms, and it was a fight that led to the predominance of the pharmaceutical industry in "modern medicine."

The controversy began in the late nineteenth century, when scientists were arguing over the concepts of monomorphism and pleomorphism. That is, whether an organism could exist in one form only or whether that organism could exist in any number of forms, depending on its context or medium. It was an important debate. Monomorphism was, at the time, the dominant trend after the introduction of the microscope and the ascendancy of Louis Pasteur—though, as early as the latter part of the nineteenth century, Carl Wilhelm von Naegeli had already insisted that there was an infinite variety of forms for any given microorganism.

Nobel Laureate Robert Koch was a major supporter of monomorphism; he specified that each disease, or type of infection, had to be the result of a specific microbial species, and he formulated criteria for physicians by which illness could be "proven," or, by studying a pathological symptom, could determine whether a patient's illness was due to the presence of microbes.

However, in subsequent years, research data emerged that bolstered the pleomorphism argument* and Koch's position on the matter came under scrutiny and was even criticized by one of his colleagues, Ernst Almquist, who said that Koch's refusal to acknowledge difference in the typhus bacillus was an attempt to, in Almquist's words, "make nature less complicated than it is." It seemed, for a time, those in the pleomorphism camp would win out, their theory of multiform organism becoming accepted fact. That's not what happened: In the end, the monomorphists, thanks to considerable political clout, won the day. Thus, the "germ theory of disease" became the new doctrine on which much of modern medicine is based. The repercussions of this victory have been far-

---

*Neisser and A. Massini, in 1906, demonstrated the bacillus coli-mutable could be converted from non–lactose fermenting to lactose fermenting; and in 1915, E. C. Hort cultivated a pleomorphic organism with both large and small rods (cocci) from patients with meningitis.

reaching. As a result, antibiotic therapy—the use of a specific drug targeted at a specific bacterial organism—became one of the fundamental principles underlying much of today's medical practice.

The use of antibiotics over the last sixty years has become widespread. However, ignored for all this time is the fact that a majority of healthy people do not develop infections. And while, of course, there is a place for appropriate antibiotics for conditions such as meningitis or surgeries like appendectomies, the integrity of a healthy immune system protects us most of the time.

But to judge from today's mainstream medical climate, you would hardly know that. Despite the prevalence of what I call the "PharmacoMafia," good health does not depend on drugs. If Dr. John Knowles, late president of the Rockefeller Foundation, was correct, 85 percent of all illnesses are the result of an unhealthy lifestyle—the end effect of unwise choices such as the use of tobacco, street drugs, and excess alcohol; inactivity; and negative attitudes. Basic lifestyle choices determine a huge majority of serious illnesses. Once the body has been devastated, medical attempts at rescue may help to prolong life, but rarely do drugs return an individual to robust health.

Additionally, in most situations, once acute illness has been stabilized, optimal residual function can be restored only with the choice of good nutrition, physical exercise, and a positive attitude. In fact, some, including me, believe that the firmest foundation for health is always attitude. You cannot afford the luxury of prolonged anger, guilt, anxiety, or depression.

Dr. Robin's provocative words challenge our entire system of medical knowledge and caution individuals to take personal responsibility for avoiding many **iatrogenic complications** (*iatrogenic*—from the Greek for "physician," *iatros,* and the suffix for "induced by," -genic—this means "physician-induced"). For instance, even though there is a general consensus among physicians regarding the proper approach to the treatment of any one medical problem, the literature itself is remarkably imperfect and even contradictory. For every article that endorses and promotes one drug, one surgical procedure, or one approach, there is likely to be another article that claims exactly the opposite. You've probably seen this in the many medical studies the media trumpets, then rescinds—coffee is good for you, coffee is bad for you; red meat prolongs life, red meat shortens life; chocolate is good for the heart, chocolate leads to high cholesterol. The list goes on.

Many of our diagnostic tests lead to disastrous results when the tests are administered in the absence of strong medical indications (symptoms) but are done primarily for the medical and legal protection of the physician. Oftentimes, the results of such tests shed no light on the medical problem and are unhelpful to the patient.

Interestingly, in his criticism of the modern medical establishment, Dr. Robin emphasizes that most physicians are wrong in their thinking about some aspect of medical care. It wasn't so long ago that bloodletting was considered a cure-all for all diseases. About 150 years ago Ignaz Philipp Semmelweis could not convince physicians that they needed to wash their hands when going from one patient to another. The incidents of puerperal fever and death went on at high rates for many years until Semmelweis proved his point by personally infecting himself and dying. Eventually physicians began at least a modicum of good sanitary practices.

An example of an iatrogenic problem that revealed that the emperor had no clothes is the estrogen and progestrin drug Prempro®. A totally illogical approach to menopause, in my opinion, that has been used for more than fifty years, Prempro® was recently revealed to be a drug far more dangerous than helpful. Most physicians ignored the fact that horse estrogen has been known to be much stronger and even much more carcinogenic than human estrogen.[8] Finally a national study was done forty years too late. Results of the negative effects of Prempro were released in the summer of 2002 in a study published in the *Journal of the American Medical Association*.[9] The medical community was "shocked" to learn just how serious these results were.

Antidepressants, another multibillion-dollar industry, have also been shown to be, in many cases, virtually useless in a number of studies.* Minimally better than placebo, some of these studies reported a complication rate of up to 25 percent. Yet the current common assumption among physicians is that antidepressant drugs are the treatment for virtually every major and minor depressive illness, despite the fact that the evidence is quite strongly against such a consensus.

These are only two examples—what I call the tip of the iceberg—of current medical system errors. I predict that eventually many other current "standards" will end up being no better than the Prempro® scandal. Other false gods of twentieth-century medicine have been abandoned with minimal public attention. Indeed, of those, only thalidomide is well known. Consider some others:

- *Radical mastectomy:* In the last fifty years there has been a remarkable controversy in medicine about the treatment

*Including I. Kirsch and T. J. Moore, "The Emperor's New Drugs: An Analysis of Antidepressant Medication Data Submitted to the U.S. Food and Drug Administration," *Prevention and Treatment* 5 (July 15, 2002): Article 23.

for breast cancer. Radical mastectomy, which is often at least severely disabling and produces many complications, has not been proven to be more effective than simple excision of breast cancer with radiation.

- *Oxygen treatment in infants:* As recently as fifty years ago, premature infants were treated with high doses of oxygen, which led to blindness.
- *Internal mammary ligation:* internal mammary ligation that was done for coronary artery disease. This turned out to be a totally useless procedure.
- *Ileal bypass for obesity:* another of the boondoggles of modern medicine, gastric stapling still exists today. This is a poor substitution for good nutrition and exercise.
- *Chloramphenicol:* Chloramphenicol was one of the antibiotics widely used back in the 1950s that led to very serious problems, including aplastic anemia. When I was an undergraduate, the chairman of Dermatology at Duke University gave me chloramphenicol for shingles despite the fact that chloramphenicol was never proven to be of any use against a virus.
- *Tonsillectomy and adenoidectomy:* These two procedures used to be prescribed almost routinely for children. There is some evidence that having these surgeries weakens the immune system forever after.
- *Psychosurgery for schizophrenia:* This procedure was not uncommon between the 1930s and 1940s, even well into the 1950s, yet it was useless and devastating to the brain and personality. Frontal lobotomy and later modifications of it were widely used for depression, ruining people forever.

- *Lumbar sympathectomy:* During the 1950s lumbar sympathectomy (destruction of the sympathetic nerve pathway to the lumbar area) was done for high blood pressure, leading to impotence and many other complications.

- *Thyroid removal and suppression:* Thyroid removal and suppression for coronary artery disease were widely done back in the 1950s to treat severe coronary artery disease—but they only made it worse.

- *Superficial femoral vein ligation:* Tying off of a superficial vein on the upper thigh was done for pulmonary embolism. Also useless.

- *Thalidomide:* One of the best-known drug disasters, of course, was the use of thalidomide. When it was given to women during pregnancy, it led to serious congenital malformations.

- *Hysterectomy:* One of the greatest errors in the medical community in the last fifty years is the widespread recommendation of hysterectomy and especially total hysterectomy (removal of the ovaries) in women. This should be reserved only for very serious problems, including cancer. Thirty-five percent of women with hysterectomies have complications.[10]

The failure of modern medicine is becoming more and more apparent every day. Indeed, I maintain that it is likely that no more than *15 percent of all illnesses* even require drugs. We have become a culture too reliant upon the medical establishment to determine our illnesses and our courses of therapy. It is ultimately your responsibility to decide what, and even whether, to seek recommended medical or surgical treatment, and to accept or reject the recommended course of action.

If you wish to age healthily and youthfully, to enjoy the benefits of the Fountain of Youth, it is your responsibility to find your way there. To get there, though, you'll have to rethink the way you look at the medical establishment.

LIFE EXPECTANCY AND THE AMERICAN MEDICAL SYSTEM

The American medical system is on the verge of collapse.[11]
—TOMMY THOMPSON,
SECRETARY OF HEALTH AND HUMAN SERVICES, 2002

If Tommy Thompson's statement is true, this could actually mean *good* news for your chances of health and longevity. Incredibly, the third leading cause of death in the United States is iatrogenic—the reported result of complications from medical treatment. Despite this fact, life expectancy of Americans has increased dramatically in the past century. (See Table 1.1.) The major reason for this increase has been an increased survival in childhood, once a very treacherous stage of life to get through. Other contributing factors include the pasteurization of milk, chlorination of water, better handling of sewage, and adequate protein intake.

Table 1.1.

COMPARING CENTURIES: LIFE EXPECTANCIES

Life Expectancy at Birth		
YEAR	MALES	FEMALES
1900	46.3	48.3
2000	74.1	79.5
Life Expectancy at Age 65		
1900	76.5	77.2
2000	81.3	84.2

Table 1.2.

**COMPARING LIFE EXPECTANCIES
AT DIFFERENT AGES**

Life Expectancy at Age 75		
YEAR	MALES	FEMALES
1900	84.5	87.1
Life Expectancy at Age 85		
1991	90.3	91.5

Table 1.3.

COMPARING LIFE EXPECTANCIES AT DIFFERENT AGES IN 1999 (MEAN AGE)

Age 20	78.7
Age 40	79.8
Age 50	79.8
Age 60	82.1

In 1991, 22 percent of all deaths occurred at age 85 or older.

Table 1.4.

LEADING CAUSES OF DEATH, ALL AGES

Heart Disease	27%
Cancer	16%
Medical Treatment	11%
Stroke	5.5%
Pneumonia and Flu	3%
Chronic Kidney Disease	3%
All Other Causes (Accidents, Suicide, Murder, Infections)	34.5%

Tables 1.1 through 1.4 are derived from National Center for Health Statistics, *Health, United States, 2004* (Hyattsville, MD).

One might guess that the increase in longevity were due to medical improvements or better medical care. This is not true— 92 percent of the factors contributing to the increase in longevity are unrelated to medical improvements. Despite many remarkable scientific discoveries over the past century, quality of life for adults has actually only improved minimally. For instance, even after a half century of the protracted "war" on cancer, life expectancy overall has increased by only four months for those who undergo chemotherapy. Quality of life for these patients has improved even less.

THE PHARMACOMAFIA

No aspect of the American medical system is more flawed than that of the drug industry (and I don't mean street drugs!). Over the past ten years, pharmaceutical companies have turned to mainstream media to advertise their products, flooding the television airwaves with commercials. The language in these commercials is often so gauzy that it is impossible to tell which condition the pill being advertised helps to ease. The United States General Accounting Office has singled out Pfizer for promulgating misleading claims for its cholesterol drug, Lipitor®, one on my list of no-no drugs (more on that later). At least 8.5 million Americans each year request and receive drugs after seeing ads for medications like Lipitor®, Flonase®, Prilosec®, and others.[12]

The *minimal* estimate for deaths from prescription drug use in the United States is 113,000 per year.[13] Other medical therapy deaths total 137,000: 12,000 deaths from surgery and 100,000 deaths from hospital errors or hospital acquired infections. Medical *treatment* is the third most likely cause of death, after heart disease and cancer. Indeed, drugs, overall—legal or illegal—are by far the greatest cause of death. The statistic can be broken down this way:

Tobacco	365,000
Alcohol	105,000
Street Drugs	56,000
Prescription Drugs	113,000
OTC (over-the-counter) Drugs	20,000+

This totals a whopping 659,000 deaths each year from drugs.

The litany of drug-related illness, disability, and death is unquestionably the greatest problem of the medical system. Since it is likely that there are more deaths from drugs than lives saved by drugs, it is critically important that informed individuals know the risks and take steps to prevent them.

Part of the reason medical care is so flawed today is that medical students are trained at med schools where most of the patients have very serious illnesses. Thus, physicians come to treat every illness as if it were life threatening. Once these students get out into the practice, most illnesses are the result of stress, certainly not requiring heroic intervention.

A visit to a physician can initiate a remarkable cascade of diagnostic and therapeutic interventions that can be dangerous to your health and life. For his part, Dr. Robin emphasizes that one should avoid hospitalization except for serious illnesses. It is my unequivocal opinion that at least 50 percent of hospital admissions even today are unnecessary. There is, perhaps, no greater flaw in the

American medical system than the concepts by which physicians start a series of diagnostic interventions. For instance, as early as the mid-1950's, it was known that physicians who used the Cornell Medical Index when diagnosing a patient could make that diagnosis with 80 percent accuracy—without any further tests. The Cornell Medical Index consists of fewer than 200 questions and involves past history, family history, and current symptoms.

But with the advent of increasingly expensive, technologically sophisticated, and potentially risky diagnostic interventions, the Cornell Medical Index has been totally abandoned—it is simply never used today.

If, after a physical exam, physicians added a comprehensive questionnaire like the Cornell Medical Index and, if they did not have a strong suspicion of some serious illness present, an invasive diagnostic test would likely not be necessary. Obviously, medical judgment is important, but medical judgment today is more often run by a concern of avoiding a medical malpractice lawsuit than it is necessarily by common sense. In addition, false positive tests are a real problem as well. There is no test, whether it is a blood test, X-ray exam, or even a pathological examination of a biopsy specimen, that is not potentially subject to false positive results. I have three women friends whose lives have been seriously traumatized by false positive mammograms leading to biopsies and, in at least one case, even the initial reading of the pathological specimen led to further severe anxiety when the ultimate diagnosis was benign. Thus, harmful practices creep into medicine and produce epidemics. The Congressional Office of Technological Assessment has concluded that well over 80 percent of all the drugs included in *Physicians' Desk Reference* (PDR) do not have adequate scientific proof to justify being there,[14] yet the number of drugs in the PDR grows exponentially every decade.

One of the great medical community errors today is the concept of a routine, periodic physical exam. In one study of 10,000 adults screened for general health, there was no difference in outcome whether they had or did not have a screening. In other words, having a "screening" evaluation, in someone with no symptoms, does not improve health or longevity. As noted earlier, false positives occur. With Pap smears, one of the most widely used diagnostic tests, two studies have shown that 40 percent of the time experts disagree on the diagnosis. As Dr. Robin concludes, "It is acceptable for a doctor to be wrong as long as all other doctors in the community are wrong in the same circumstance."[15]

There is a great oversupply of physicians in the United States, probably twice as many as we need. The incidence of medical complications and iatrogenic death is directly related to this oversupply. I strongly support the concept that virtually all primary medical care should be done by holistically oriented nurse practitioners, not general physicians.

Thus, one of the requirements for extending life beyond 100 is: *Avoid medical care that is not essential to life or function.*

2

STRESS AND DISTRESS: RESTORING HUMAN DNA FOR HEALTH AND LONGEVITY

THE CONCEPT AND
PHYSIOLOGY OF STRESS

In 1999 both *Time* and *Esquire* selected *Faster: The Acceleration of Just About Everything*, by James Gleick, as the book of the year.[16] Gleick's book is a delightful spoof on our society's eat-and-run, sex-and-paperwork existence. "Never in the history of the human race," he writes, "have so many had so much to do in so little time."[17] He also quotes Meher Baba, an Indian mystic: "A mind that is fast is sick. A mind that is slow is sound. A mind that is still is divine."[18]

Dr. Hans Selye is widely recognized as the "father" of the concept of stress. In 1926, during his second year of medical school,

Selye began developing his famous theories of the influence of stress on the human ability to cope with and adapt to pressures of injury and disease. He discovered that a wide variety of diseases present with very similar symptoms, which he called the "stress syndrome," or the "general adaptation syndrome."[19]

The theory was that, essentially, stress may impact any individual from many different points of "entry," and that any excess pressure can cause a stress reaction in the body. This pressure may be physical in nature (e.g., temperature or trauma), chemical (e.g., alcohol), emotional (e.g., anger, depression), electromagnetic (e.g., 60 cycle), or nuclear (radiation).

The body's response to stress is a chain reaction of sorts. The beginning of the reaction occurs in the pituitary gland, which releases a hormone called ACTH (adrenocorticotrophic hormone). With many stressors, the autonomic nervous system, specifically the sympathetic system, is activated simultaneously. The sympathetic nervous system releases **norepinephrine (NE)**, or "adrenaline," which is a further stimulus announcing an alarm.

With the pituitary secreting ACTH, the adrenal gland, in reaction, then secretes cortisol. The cortisol raises blood sugar levels, which, in turn, engineers a release of insulin from the pancreas. The release of cortisol also affects the thymus gland and the entire lymph system, as well as white blood cells and the stomach. Selye considered this initial response to be an "alarm reaction" to a stressor.

As dire as the alarm reaction sounds, Selye emphasized that most of us adapt to a new stress. Take coffee, for example. Let's say someone who has never had a cup of coffee in his life decides to pour himself a cup and see what all the fuss is about. That first cup will result in a doubling of the output of NE, a neurotransmitter. In fact, for that neophyte coffee drinker, his NE level won't return to normal for some thirty-six hours. But if the individual drinks a cup of coffee every day, after a week or so, the morning java will have no significant effect upon NE or cortisol levels. He has adapted to the stress of the introduction of coffee into the system. The same is true for cigarettes. That first, ill-advised cigarette creates an alarm reaction resulting in roughly the same output of NE and cortisol as with the coffee. But, again, as the individual smokes more and more cigarettes, an adaption occurs. These two examples deviate, interestingly, in the recovery time necessary for the adaption: NE returns to baseline level after only fifteen to twenty minutes after that first cigarette.

Selye also demonstrated that subliminal or subthreshold levels of stress are cumulative. Therefore, one-third of a cigarette or one-third of a cup of coffee would not initially induce a stress response, but if you put all those together you will elicit an "alarm reaction."

The adaptation to stress isn't a neat affair. Numerous cascade effects take place as the body adapts to the stressor. For instance, when cortisol levels are raised in reaction to some type of stress, the adrenal gland releases the hormone DHEA (dehydroepiandrosterone) to bring that cortisol level back to normal. (One of the earliest signs of adrenal burnout or overload is a gradual decrease in DHEA levels.) This decrease begins for most individuals after the age of thirty. (An entire section of this chapter will be devoted to DHEA.)

As we've seen, a little stress leads to changes to physiology—which the body fairly promptly corrects, putting it back into balance. But, although the human body is capable of adapting to an astonishing variety of stressors, there are times when it cannot adapt. When this happens, various symptoms begin to appear.

There are, essentially, roughly 150 symptoms that indicate an inability to adapt to stress, and the reaction appears to be extremely individualized. As total stress increases, the total number of symptoms also increases. By the time one gets to twenty or more symptoms, adrenal overload is occurring, and the DHEA level is already beginning to be less than optimal. At about that same time, the pancreas's ability to respond to all the ups and downs of stress stimulation and the release of cortisol also becomes inefficient.

One critically important result of this reaction is an increased resistance to insulin, and an inappropriate release of insulin—leading first to hypoglycemia, and eventually to burnout of the pancreas or even adult-onset diabetes. This is inevitably accompanied by a decrease in IGF-1 (**insulinlike growth hormone factor-1**). This particular hormone decreases significantly as stress increases. Two of the most important measurements, then, of burnout are lower levels of DHEA and lower levels of IGF-1.

One of the basic physiological reactions of life is oxidation. We breathe to bring in oxygen, and we burn sugar in one form or another for energy. As the stress response and maladaptation occur, the ability of the body to promote homeostasis, or return to normal internal balance, decreases and we wind up with increasing numbers of chemical compounds called free radicals. Free radicals are the result of a weak chemical bond—when those bonds split, free radicals are formed. They are unstable—wild cards—and in their effort to gain stability, by trying to find an electron, they attack stable molecules in order to take those molecules' electrons. What this translates into, for people unfortunate enough to have high levels of free radicals in their system, is an attack on body tissue. Ultimately, it is the free radicals that cause aging, disease, and death. And it is all due to stress.

Therefore, if we can keep our DHEA levels at a healthy optimal level, our IGF-1 (a reflection of a healthy immune system) at a healthy optimal level, and our free radicals at the lowest possible level, our body will actually regenerate itself and rejuvenate itself for an indefinite period of time. Leonard Orr, for instance, believes that this period of time could be hundreds of years.[20]

While most scientists do not believe in such indefinite life expectancy, Orr is not alone in his belief. Many scientists have long felt it possible to increase one's life expectancy by a number of years during one's own life span. This concept was originally introduced by Dr. Roy Walford.[21] His work emphasized reducing caloric intake significantly as a means of living "120 years or more." There are two experiments currently in progress to determine if caloric restriction extends life span in monkeys.[22] The most recent results, reported by J. A. Mattison and colleagues from the National Institute on Aging, reveal that a 30 percent reduction in caloric intake "suggests that CR [calorie restriction] will have beneficial effects on morbidity and mortality." Virtually every physiological aspect of aging is slowed in these monkeys who have been observed for over eighteen years.[23]

Sounds simple. Fewer calories, longer life. The problem with this suggestion to reduce caloric intake is that people aren't taking it. As the message gets louder and louder, we grow more and more deaf. We are experiencing an obesity epidemic. People are not eating 30 percent fewer calories than optimal; they are eating 30 percent more than optimal! Of course the PharmacoMafia experts have long been attempting to develop a pill which will mimic calorie cutting.

In particular, drug companies are looking at a compound called resveratrol that is found in the skin of grapes, and ingested mainly in the form of red wine. Many people believe that a good part of the reason the French can eat gobs more fat than Americans eat, while maintaining a lower incidence of heart disease, is their significant intake of red wine. I predict that the creation of calorie-limiting drugs will cause many more complications than benefits and will probably shorten life and not extend it. But time will tell. In the meantime, the most effective tool for health that you can use is the reduction of stress in your own life. There are several ways to accomplish this, which are explored in the next chapter. In the meantime, let's turn our attention to DHEA.

DHEA (DEHYDROEPIANDROSTERONE)

I consider DHEA, the most abundant hormone in the human body, also to be the single most important chemical in evaluating health and longevity. As with most hormones, it is manufactured from cholesterol in the body through an intermediary called **pregnenolone**, either directly into DHEA or through conversion to **progesterone** into DHEA. Progesterone is a building block of cortisol and aldosterone, the hormone that controls water and potassium metabolism. Progesterone is also a precursor of estrogen and testosterone. DHEA may be converted into estrogen and testosterone but, more important, it is a major feedback modulator of all hormones in the body.

DHEA levels are important gauges for human health. Levels of DHEA are found to be low or deficient in nearly every major disease, including anxiety, autoimmune disorders, cancer, coronary artery disease, depression, diabetes, high blood pressure, obesity, various immune dysfunctions, and more.

Just as Dr. Selye demonstrated progression from alarm to adaptation to maladaptation to degeneration and exhaustion or burnout, it is my impression that this progression is highly correlated with DHEA levels. (See Figure 2.1, DHEA Levels and Stress.) In my experience, 100 percent of several thousand patients tested at my clinic have DHEA levels that are, at best, fair to low, and 50 percent of patients are in serious deficiency no matter what the disease. As we might expect, high levels of DHEA are correlated with optimal levels of growth hormone, especially IGF-1, an insulinlike promoter of growth. The major contributor to decreased growth hormone and low levels of IGF-1 is obesity.

DHEA LEVELS AND STRESS

SERIOUS DEFICIENCY	WORRISOME LOW	FAIR	GOOD	EXCELLENT
Male <180	180–349	350–599	600–749	750–1250
Female <130	130–299	300–449	450–549	550–980
Exhaustion	← Progressive Maladaptation		Adaptation	Homeostasis
↓	↓			
Serious Illness	Degeneration			

Figure 2.1

Any metabolic pathway that enhances homeostasis is likely to be beneficial in helping individuals avoid burnout and maintain optimal levels of DHEA. For instance, growth hormone is enhanced by increased intake of **arginine** and **ornithine**. **Tyrosine** and **phenylalanine** are the foundations for making norepinephrine and, in the short run, a little norepinephrine helps stimulate the release of DHEA. However, accelerated amounts of norepinephrine eventually depress DHEA.

There are also many drugs that interfere with DHEA, one of the most common being propranolol, a drug that blocks normal adrenal production of norepinephrine. This drug, and others like it, are called **beta-blockers**, sometimes prescribed by doctors for high blood pressure or to treat anxiety or panic disorders. Beta-blockers, as well as calcium channel blockers, have negative effects on DHEA levels.

A major antioxidant that helps to decrease free radicals, DHEA is a major indicator of overall health and a strong immune system. The most important metabolic effects and elements of DHEA include:

- Stabilization of glucose metabolism
- Regulation of all hormones
- Decreasing of cholesterol levels
- The precursor of estrogen and testosterone
- Assistance of homeostasis after the stress reaction
- Enhancement of immune function
- Maintenance of youth and health
- Stabilization of weight

Perhaps more than any other question, I am asked whether one should take an oral DHEA supplement. My answer is: only rarely. Oral DHEA may exacerbate latent cancer of the breast, ovary, uterus, and prostate.[24] However, individuals who have serious illnesses such as heart disease, rheumatoid arthritis, lupus, multiple sclerosis or serious infections; are having major surgery; or who are in other such serious acute or chronic situations may well benefit from oral doses of DHEA, under the most extreme circumstances as much as 1,000 mg. a day. However, you should never take this on your own, only under a doctor's supervision. Also, it should ordinarily only be taken during the acute treatment phase. Fortunately, there are four excellent techniques for restoring DHEA naturally, which I outline below, and I strongly recommend these.

If you have ever taken oral DHEA for an acute medical situation, or even if you have taken it thinking it was a good idea, you should wean yourself off it over a period of three to four months while adding as many of the following techniques outlined below as possible. After you have withdrawn from the DHEA, cutting down slowly over a minimum period of one month, continue with the techniques for at least another month and then recheck your DHEA blood or salivary level. If your level is above the lower limit of normal, continue with the restoration procedure.

Natural enhancement of DHEA has been reported with physical exercise, various stress-reduction programs, meditation, and caloric restriction. DHEA is significantly higher in ten- to sixteen-year-old athletes compared to nonathletes, just as testosterone, growth hormone, cortisol, and bone age (bone strength) are also greater in athletes. In other words, exercise accelerates bone age. In addition, these other neurochemical responses to maturing are also greater in athletes.

DHEA levels in consistent meditators are comparable to those of nonmeditators who are *five to ten years younger.* An active sex life also seems to be essential for optimal levels of DHEA, and there is some evidence that even sexual fantasy helps to raise DHEA levels. Sunshine and being outside in natural light are also enhancers of DHEA.

THE RINGS OF LIFE

Over the past ten years, I have discovered in the human body five circuits that activate specific chemical pathways. I call them the Five Sacred Rings: they are energetic circuits that specifically optimize DHEA, neurotensin, calcitonin, and aldosterone and markedly reduce free radicals. Useful techniques for stimulating the Five Sacred Rings can be found below. (See **Technique #4**, page 58.)

THE RING OF FIRE

Electrical stimulation of the **Ring of Fire** significantly raises DHEA an average of 60 percent and up to 100 percent or more. This should be done with a **SheLi TENS™**, a safe electrical stimulator that includes the frequencies of 54 to 78 billion cycles per second, those natural resonant frequencies of DNA.* Using knowledge of the meridians and acupuncture points of traditional Chinese medicine, I have determined that stimulation of specific acupuncture points—and their corresponding organs—will raise the level of DHEA. You start with the points at the bottom of the body and work up toward the top. As you sense the energetic circuit, the energy moves from the

---

*I have only stimulated the Five Sacred Ring points using the SheLi TENS™ and the Liss stimulator, not with needles, and this has proven a successful tactic. While the Liss is superior for transcranial stimulation, I have found it is somewhat less effective when used on the Ring points. The SheLi TENS™, on the other hand, which has the Giga frequencies of DNA, is the best stimulator for activation of the Rings. The sketches of the five rings are taken from *The Science of Medical Intuition* by Caroline M. Myss and C. Norman Shealy, published by Sounds True (Boulder, CO), 2002. Reprinted here by permission.

ankles up to the top of the head, and from the top of the head back down to the ankles in a continuous flow of energy. It is called "fire" because DHEA is the single most important indication of your energetic fire—it's the battery of your life energy.

See below and Figure 2.2 for the location of these twelve points. They are called: **Kidney K3 (bilateral), Conception Vessel CV2, Conception Vessel CV6, Bladder B22 (bilateral), Conception Vessel CV18, Master of the Heart MH6 (bilateral), Large Intestine LI18 (bilateral), and Governing Vessel GV20.**[25]

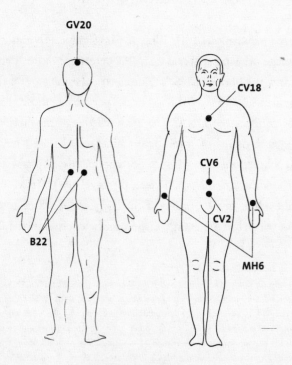

THE RING OF FIRE

THE RING OF FIRE

K3 *(Kidney)* Midway between the tip of the medial malleolus and the tendo calcaneus

CV2 *(Conception Vessel)* in the superior border of the pubic syphonis, in the middle of the abdomen

CV6 *(Conception Vessel)* 1.5 cun below the umbilicus in the middle of the abdomen

B22 *(Bladder)* 1.5 cun lateral to the lower border of the spinous process of the first lumbar vertebra

MH6 *(Master of the Heart)* On the ulnar side of the wrist, on the radial side of the tendon M. flexor carpi ulnaris, below the pisiform bone

LI18 *(Large Intestine)* 3 cun lateral to the thyroid cartilage, between the sternal, head, and the clavicular head of the sternocleitidomastoid muscle

CV18 *(Conception Vessel)* is on the midline of the sternum 1.6 cun above the line of the two nipples, at the level of the third intercostal rib

GV20 *(Governing Vessel)* 7 cun above the posterior hairline, midway on a line connecting the apex of both ears

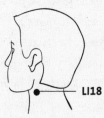

LI18

K3 (BILATERAL)

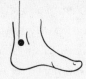

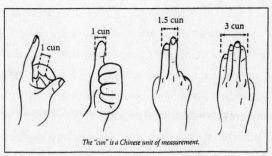

The "cun" is a Chinese unit of measurement.

Figure 2.2

In addition to the Ring of Fire, four other circuits are important in maintaining health and establishing longevity:

THE RING OF AIR

Electrical stimulation of the **Ring of Air** increases neurotensin, an endogenous tridecapeptide found in the central nervous system. It is a neurotransmitter that is produced in the hypothalamus, amygdala, basal ganglia, dorsal gray of the spinal cord, and in the intestine itself. It plays a very major role in pain perception, but its analgesic effects are not blocked by opioid antagonists. It also affects pituitary hormone release and gastrointestinal activity. Two possible aspects of neurotensin in the central nervous system are its involvement in the etiology of schizophrenia and its analgesic properties. Neurotensin actually is antipsychotic so that, theoretically, enhancing neurotensin could prevent or treat schizophrenia. Neurotensin also affects pituitary hormone regulation in a remarkable variety of gastrointestinal functions, especially metabolism of fat. Neurotensin is neuroleptic, not in the pharmaceutical sense of the word but in its ability to allow cognitive dissociation. That is, neurotensin essentially increases the ability of an individual to detach from physical sensation yet be mentally quite alert.[26] There is considerable clinical evidence of antinociceptive, or pain-relieving, benefits of neurotensin. In nature, however, it is relatively rapidly metabolized, so that giving neurotensin externally, either orally or by injection, is not therapeutically feasible. At low-blood sugar levels, neurotensin stimulates release of insulin. Interestingly, release of glucagons and somatostatin, the normal neurochemicals that are stimulated by glucose or arginine, is inhibited by neurotensin. There is a close metabolic relationship between neurotensin and histamine, with neurotensin effects being reversed by histamine-receptive blocks.

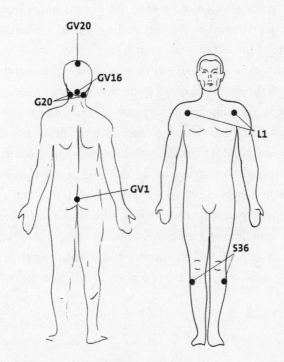

THE RING OF AIR

The Ring of Air points are (see Figure 2.3): Spleen 1A (bilateral), Liver 3 (bilateral), Stomach 36 (bilateral), Lung 1 (bilateral), Gall Bladder 20, Governing Vessel 1, Governing Vessel 16, Governing Vessel 20 (bilateral).

In summary, neurotensin has anti-inflammatory properties and decreases the body's response to all known causes of inflammation. Because of its short half-life, an internally activated production is the most effective way of enhancing neurotensin effect. It seems quite likely, considering the benefits of neurotensin and in our early clinical experiences with it, that stimulation of the Ring of Air increases emotional mental detachment and helps stimulate holographic thinking or intuition. I have done visualization and massage of these specific thirteen acupuncture points in classroom settings with hundreds of individuals, most of whom report subjective feelings of increased connectedness accomplished at the highest levels of meditative experience. There is no way of measuring lucidity or meditative states of awareness, and obviously much more clinical work needs to be done, both to determine the subjective effects of activation of the Ring of Air as well as other implications from increased levels of neurotensin. From a theoretical point of view, stimulation of the Ring of Air could be of some benefit in tinnitus and hearing loss. Stimulation of the Ring of Air with the SheLi TENS™ has increased neurotensin levels as much as 1,150 percent with an average increase of 300 percent.

THE RING OF AIR

SP1A *(Spleen)* on the medial side of the big toe, 0.1 cun posterior to the corner of the nail

LIV3 *(Liver)* between the first and second toe, 2 cun proximal to the margin of the web

S36 *(Stomach)* 3 cun below the lateral side of the patella, one finger breadth from the anterior crest of the tibia

LI *(Lung)* on the lateral aspect of the chest, in the interspace of the first and second ribs, 6 cun lateral to the midline of the chest

G20 *(Gall Bladder)* in the depression between the M. sternocleidomastoid and the upper portion of the M. trapezius; specifically, between the depression directly inferior to the occipital protuberance and the mastoid

GV1 *(Governing Vessel)* tip of the coccyx

GV16 *(Governing Vessel)* directly below the occipital protuberance, in the midline, in a depression 1 cun above the hairline

GV20 *(Governing Vessel)* 7 cun above the posterior hairline, midway on a line connecting the apex of both ears

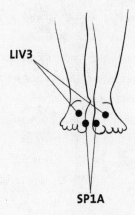

LIV3

SP1A

Figure 2.3

THE RING OF WATER

Electrical stimulation of the thirteen points of the **Ring of Water** increases aldosterone, the adrenal hormone that regulates water and mineral metabolism. Interestingly, stimulation of the Ring of

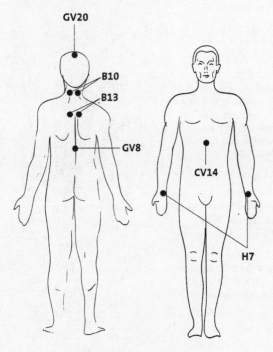

THE RING OF WATER

The points of the Ring of Water are (see Figure 2.4): Spleen 4 (bilateral), Heart 7 (bilateral), Bladder 10 (bilateral), Bladder 13 (bilateral), Conception Vessel 14, Triple Heater 16 (bilateral), Governing Vessel 8, Governing Vessel 20.

Water optimizes aldosterone levels. Low levels of aldosterone are more likely in the elderly who are prone to problems with water metabolism. One of the additional benefits of stimulating the Ring of Water may be improved emotional balance. Also, when combining stimulation of the Ring of Water with stimulation of the Ring of Fire, I have found significant weight loss.

THE RING OF WATER

SP4 *(Spleen)* on the medial aspect of the foot, in a depression at the anterior and inferior border of the first metatarsal bone, at the junction of the "red and white" skin

H7 *(Heart)* on the ulnar side of the wrist, on the posterior border of the pisiform bone, in the depression at the radial side of the tendon M. flexor carpi ulnaris

B10 *(Bladder)* 1.3 cun lateral to midline of 1st and 2nd cervical vertebrae, on the lateral side of M. trapezius

B13 *(Bladder)* 1.5 cun lateral to the lower border of the spinos process of the third thoracic vertebra

CV14 *(Conception Vessel)* 6 cun above the umbilicus, on the midline of the abdomen

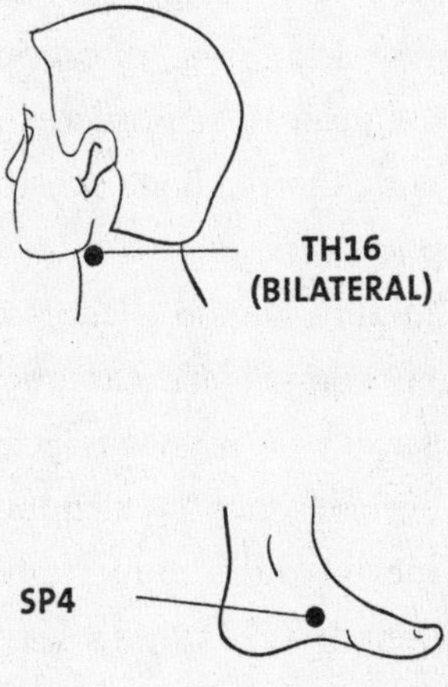

Figure 2.4

TH16 *(Triple Healer)* posterior and inferior to the mastoid process, in the posterior border at M. sternocleidomastoid, at the level of the angle of the mandible

GV8 *(Governing Vessel)* below the spinous process of the ninth thoracic vertebra

GV20 *(Governing Vessel)* 7 cun above the posterior hairline, midway on a line connecting the apex of both ears

The Ring of Earth

Stimulation of the **Ring of Earth** with the SheLi TENS™ increases calcitonin levels within one hour of initial stimulation. **Calcitonin** was discovered in 1961 and has been widely used clinically for the treatment of Paget's disease, hypercalcimia, osteoporosis, and for relief of bone pain. Calcitonin is a hormone produced by the thyroid gland and is secreted in response to high levels of calcium in the blood. It lowers the level of calcium by inhibiting bone resorption or the dissolution of bone tissue. Calcitonin plays a role in pain relief and has been noted for its analgesic effects in bone metastases in a variety of cancers, as well as in phantom-limb pain. It also enhances or produces recalcification of osteopenic bone (that with lowered bone density) and has been used for treatment of peptic ulcers.

Clinically, salmon calcitonin is the form widely used therapeutically, but injected pharmaceutical-grade calcitonin from the salmon has a small risk of anaphylactic shock, which can be fatal. However, even this salmon calcitonin is a powerful analgesic agent with a potency of thirty to fifty times that of morphine, milligram for milligram. In 1992 world sales of calcitonin exceeded $900 million, of which 85 percent was given for osteoporosis.

Osteoporosis is thinning of the bone through reduction in bone mass due to depletion of calcium and bone protein. Osteoporosis predisposes individuals to fractures, which are often slow to heal and heal poorly. Hip fractures are most common, especially in older adults, particularly postmenopausal women, patients using steroids, and those taking many different steroidal drugs as well as over-the-

counter nonsteroidal anti-inflammatory drugs. Unchecked, osteoporosis can lead to changes in posture, physical abnormality (particularly in the form of a hunchback, known commonly as "dowager's
hump"), and decreased mobility. The Food and Drug Administration (FDA) has approved a salmon calcitonin in nasal spray form, as
well as the injectable form for treatment of osteoporosis. However,
the nasal spray may cause ulceration, inflammation of the nose or
rhinitis, nosebleeds, and even sinusitis.

The effect of space travel on calcitonin levels has been the subject of studies both in animals and astronauts, and it is quite well
demonstrated that even short space flights disrupt calcium metabolism and lead to decreased blood calcitonin levels as well as to
rapid onset of bone loss. Interestingly, salmon calcitonin has been
more effective than indomethacin in preventing heterotopic ossifi-
cation (deposits of calcium leading to bone formation outside the
skeleton itself). Calcitonin has also been seen to help osteopenia
(lowered bone density) as well as the pain in juvenile idiopathic
arthritis.

Nonosteoporotic vertebral fractures (i.e., not from osteoporosis) have been quite successfully treated with calcitonin, with the
pain being reduced rapidly, also having the pain relief allow earlier
mobilization and gradual restoration of activity. Hip fracture is a
leading cause of death in the elderly; thus stimulation of the Ring
of Earth appears to have a major potential for maintaining long-
term health and longevity, as well as providing pain relief. It
should also be considered for astronauts.

One of the most interesting effects of calcitonin is in treatment
of chronic phantom-limb pain, that is, the pain that is sometimes
totally incapacitating after amputation of a limb. In a study of cal-

citonin versus cimetidine in gastric ulcers, it was reported that the calcitonin group had some mild side effects of headache, nausea, and vomiting, but calcitonin was a superior antiulcer drug.

Given the fact that electrical stimulation of the thirteen Ring of Earth acupuncture points can raise calcitonin by **over** 80 percent, this appears to be a very natural and safe approach without the risk

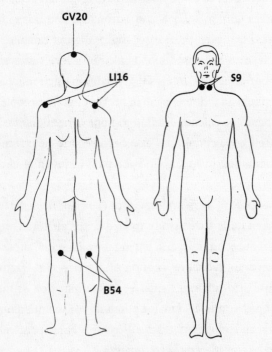

THE RING OF EARTH

The points of the Ring of Earth are (see Figure 2.5): Kidney 1 (bilateral), Bladder 54 (bilateral), Bladder 60 (bilateral), Small Intestine 17, Stomach 9, Large Intestine 16, Governing Vessel 20.

of the pharmaceutically available salmon calcitonin. At least it is the Ring of Earth that causes the human calcitonin to be produced in that particular human's body!

It is essential that thyroid function be reasonably good in order to activate calcitonin. Thus, you should check your metabolic rate by measuring your morning temperature at least several mornings before you get out of bed. If your oral temperature with the thermometer held in the mouth at least three to five minutes is below 97.6° F, you have subclinical hypothyroidism. You should take 1,500 to 2,000 mcg. of iodine daily for one to two months and see if you bring your temperature up to normal. If not, I would recommend continuing to take the iodine for at least another two months while daily stimulating the Ring of Fire. Most people who are on thyroid-replacement therapy are going to have low or totally depleted levels of calcitonin. I am not certain that stimulating the Ring of Earth will raise calcitonin when the thyroid is suppressed by taking thyroid medication. This is true whether one is taking the synthetic thyroid medication or animal-derived thyroid. Obviously, those individuals who have had a surgical removal of the thyroid gland have no known mechanism for producing calcitonin, and stimulation of the Ring of Earth in them may not benefit.

THE RING OF CRYSTAL

When I received the intuitive flash that led to the **Ring of Crystal,** I sensed that this is the crucial circuit for *regeneration* of the nervous system and the body as a whole. Cellular physiologists tell us that every cell in the body is regenerated within a maximum of

THE SCIENCE OF MEDICAL INTUITION

THE RING OF EARTH

K1 *(Kidney)* In the depression at the junction of anterior and middle third of the sole in a depression between the 2nd and 3rd metatarso-phalangeal joint when the toes are plantar flexed

B54 *(Bladder)* Exact midpoint of the popliteal transverse crease

B60 *(Bladder)* Between the posterior border of the external malleolus and the medial aspect of tendo calcaneus at the same level as the tip of the malleolus

LI16 *(Large intestine)* In the depression between the clavico-acromal extremity and the spine of the scapulae

ST9 *(Stomach)* Posterior to the common carotid artery on the anterior border of the M. Sternocleidomastoid, lateral to the thyroid cartilage

SI17 *(Small intestine)* Posterior to the angle of the jaw on the anterior border of M. sternocleidomastoid

GV20 *(Governing vessel)* 7 cun above the posterior hairline, midway on a line connecting apex of both ears

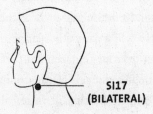

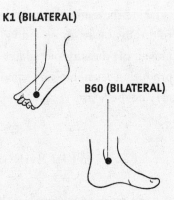

Figure 2.5

seven years. Some cells, of course, are replaced within hours or days. Unfortunately, it is free radicals that ultimately adversely affect cell physiology and regeneration.

Free radicals are somewhat like the ozone layer, which is essential in destroying some cosmic radiation and provides a protective atmospheric shield. In our bodies, free radicals are "wild" oxidized chemicals that contribute to virtually all illnesses, aging, and death.

Stimulation of the Ring of Crystal, which reduces free radicals, appears either to enhance natural antioxidant levels or to allow the body to produce its own antioxidants.

Oxidative stress is thought to be involved in the aging process in aerobic organisms and to play a role in the pathogenesis of a variety of disease states, including Alzheimer's disease, myocardial infarction, arteriosclerosis, Parkinson's, autoimmune diseases, radiation injury, emphysema, sunburn, glomerular disorders, schizophrenia, sickle cell disease, leukemia, osteoporosis, infertility, cancer, retinopathy, and noise-related hearing impairment. Oxidative stress is the result of free radicals (e.g., the hydroxyl radical) reacting with biological macromolecules such as lipids, proteins, nucleic acid, and carbohydrates. The initial reaction generates a second radical, which in turn can react with a second macromolecule to continue the chain reaction. In the process of reacting, a free radical can modify protein or DNA structures, disrupt individual nucleotide bases, and thereby cause effects such as single-strand breaks and cross-linking in nucleic acids—that is, in our DNA!

Free-radical-induced oxidative stress is a major factor in the long-term tissue degradation associated with aging. Aging appears to be the cumulative result of oxidative damage to the cells and tissues of the body that arises primarily as the result of aerobic metabolism or burning oxygen. Several lines of evidence have been used to support this hypothesis including the claims that:

- variation in the life span of different species is correlated with metabolic rate and protective antioxidant activity.
- enhanced expression of antioxidant enzymes in experimental animals can produce a significant increase in longevity.
- cellular levels of free-radical damage increase with age.
- reduced caloric intake leads to a decline in the production of free radicals and an increase in life span.

The free-radical theory may also be used to explain many of the structural features that develop with aging, including the lipid peroxidation of membranes, the formation of age pigments, cross-linkage of proteins, DNA damage, and decline of mitochondrial function. Most free-radical damage is in the cholesterol/lipid structure of the body. Thus, lipids that have been converted into free radicals are the results of lipid peroxidation.

Free radicals occur in trace quantities in biological tissues and are extremely reactive. Because of the difficulty of directly measuring free radicals in living individuals, measurements can be made using biomarkers, for example, an assay of antioxidant vitamins and free radical scavengers. Therefore, oxidative stress has been mainly observed through indirect biomarkers in aerobic organisms such as measuring oxidative damage to tissues and organs. Such damage is prevented by a network of defenses, which include antioxidant and repairing enzymes as well as small molecules with scavenging ability, for example, antioxidant vitamins. For these reasons, the assay of antioxidant vitamins and of small molecular free-radical scavengers in biological milieus may be used, if appropriately performed, to quantify the defense status against oxidative damage and to provide an indirect estimate of free-radical production in aging individuals.

Malondialdehyde (MDA) levels in both blood and urine have been among the most widely used free-radical markers. Measurement of MDA excretion in the urine became available in 1964. MDA is the end product of lipid peroxidation, and this urinary colorimetric assay represents by far the simplest approach to measurement of free-radical activity. Furthermore, this colorimetric assay has been highly significantly correlated with the more sophisticated fluorometric laboratory approach.

Mammalian cells normally possess elaborate defense mechanisms to detoxify radicals. Free-radical-scavenging antioxidants such as vitamin C, vitamin E, and beta-carotene interrupt the chain by capturing the radical. Excessive amounts of cellular oxidants, which animal cells constantly produce, can induce oxidative damage. Cellular antioxidants provide a defense against the damaging effects of the cellular oxidants. However, in moderate concentrations, cellular oxidants are necessary for a number of protective reactions that eliminate cancerous and other life-threatening cells such as antimicrobial phagocytosis (ingestion of cells) and apoptosis (destruction of cells from within). Abundant antioxidants could suppress normal protective functions, especially in people with low baseline levels of cellular oxidants. Conventional antioxidant supplements can be harmful in high doses, and safe antioxidant supplementation requires an accurate dosage level according to each individual's needs.

A delicate balance exists between the production of free radicals and the production of antioxidants. Free radicals are produced in the body as by-products of normal metabolism, as well as being a result of exposure to radiation and some environmental pollutants. They are normally neutralized by the body's production of antioxidant enzymes (super oxide dismutase, catalase, and glutathion peroxidase) and the nutrient-derived antioxidant small molecules such as vitamin A, vitamin C, carotene, flavonoids, glutathione, uric acid, and taurine. The natural balance can be upset by pathological conditions in which there is increased oxidative stress, such as diabetes. Oxidative stress can cause a reduction in the body's normal production of antioxidant enzymes.

Despite extensive research on the use of antioxidant supplements, however, there is no clear-cut consensus that these antioxidants are totally successful in reducing or eliminating free radicals. There is, however, considerable evidence that the antioxidants found in natural sources, such as vegetables and fruits, do have a beneficial effect. It is of considerable interest that antioxidants themselves do not ordinarily cross the blood-brain barrier, a significant problem in reducing the known negative effects of free radicals in many degenerative central-nervous-system diseases such as Alzheimer's.

Interestingly, there is only one known nonantioxidant technique for reducing free radicals: that is, six degrees head-down bed rest. However, that can require as much as seventeen days of simulated weightlessness. Furthermore, bed rest and the corresponding inactivity have also been linked to increased free-radical levels.

The discovery that stimulation of the Ring of Crystal markedly reduces free radicals is the first major new breakthrough in our search for health and longevity. Every human should take advantage of this remarkable innovation. In 80 percent of individuals, free radicals are reduced an average of 80 percent after just two to three days of stimulation of the Ring of Crystal. Indeed, in at least 50 percent of individuals, free radicals are eliminated. Considering all the aspects of managing free radicals and the pathology associated with them, the discovery of a significant decrease in

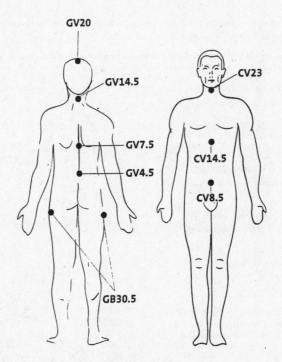

THE RING OF CRYSTAL

The points of the Ring of Crystal are (see Figure 2.6): Spleen 4 (bilateral), Gall Bladder 30.5 (bilateral), Conception Vessel 8.5, Governing Vessel 4.5, Conception Vessel 14.5, Governing Vessel 7.5, Governing Vessel 14.5, Conception Vessel 23, Gall Bladder 11, Governing Vessel 20.

free radicals after electrical stimulation of the Ring of Crystal is of great interest. A patent has been granted.

Ideally, all rings should be stimulated with the SheLi TENS™.

THE RING OF CRYSTAL

SP4 *(Spleen)* on the medial aspect of the foot, in a depression at the anterior and inferior borders of first metatarsal bone, at the juncture of the "red and white" skin

GB30.5 *(Gall Bladder)* 2 cun lateral of the greater trochanter to the major trochanter, lateral side of the upper leg

CV8.5 *(Conception Vessel)* .5 cun above the umbilicus

GV4.5 *(Governing Vessel)* on the spinous process of the 2nd lumbar vertebra

CV14.5 *(Conception Vessel)* 6.5 cun above the umbilicus on the midline of the abdomen

GV7.5 *(Governing Vessel)* on the spinous process of the ninth thoracic vertebra

GV14.5 *(Governing Vessel)* on the spinous process of the third cervical vertebra

CV23 *(Conception Vessel)* midline of the neck, midway between the tip of the cricoid cartilage and the border of the mandible

GB11 *(Gall Bladder)* in the depression 1 cun posterior of the horizontal line of the auricle

GV20 *(Governing Vessel)* 7 cun above the posterior hairline, midway on a line connecting the apex of both ears

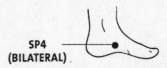

Figure 2.6

TECHNIQUES FOR INCREASING DHEA LEVELS

TECHNIQUE #1

The simplest technique for raising DHEA is taking a combination of 2 grams of vitamin C, 1 gram of methylsulphonylmethane, 6 mg. of beta 1,3 glucan, and 60 mcg. of molybdenum. This is found in four capsules of Dr. sHEALy's Youth Formula™. I strongly recommend this for all adults. This raises DHEA an average of 60 percent.

TECHNIQUE #2

The next in ease is the use of **transdermal magnesium,** and the magnesium component will be discussed in greater detail (after Technique #4). At least three teaspoons a day of Dr. sHEALy's Biogenics® Magnesium Lotion applied to the skin raise both DHEA and intracellular magnesium levels an average of 60 percent.

TECHNIQUE #3

One quarter teaspoon of natural progesterone cream twice a day applied to the skin raises DHEA an average of 60 percent. Premenopausal women should use natural progesterone only from days ten to twenty-eight of their cycle.

TECHNIQUE #4: STIMULATION OF
THE FIVE SACRED RINGS

I strongly recommend that all individuals begin regular stimulation of three of the Five Sacred Rings no later than age fifty. The sequence ought to be Fire, Earth, Crystal, and twice weekly. That is, one would stimulate only one ring a day and would be able to make two complete circuits and be able to do all three rings twice each week with one day off. It is this approach and the good health habits outlined throughout this book that offer the potential for living healthily to 140 years of age! Attitude remains the most important determinant of health. With an attitude of *health* and *longevity*, as well as stimulation of the rings, you really are the creator of your reality! Incidentally, although I have not personally used acupuncture on the rings, one of my students has done a study with acupuncture needles, activating the Ring of Crystal. Her results demonstrated far less of a decrease in free radicals than those I have consistently achieved with the Ring of Crystal.

Currently I am investigating the potential of stimulating only two points for increasing DHEA and calcitonin, while lowering free radicals. If this can be achieved, increased human longevity will be increased with minimal effort. I simply apply the SheLi TENS™ while I do my morning exercise.

Using all these techniques together, DHEA increases much more than using any one of them alone. For those with the lowest levels of DHEA, I strongly recommend that you use all four of these techniques, as well as increase exercise, get outside more, and enjoy a healthy sex life!

MAGNESIUM

Magnesium deficiency may be more common than any other chemical or nutritional deficiency. At least the third most prevalent mineral in the human body, magnesium is a natural calcium channel blocker. This means that there is a synergistic relationship between calcium and magnesium. (Magnesium is concentrated inside cells and calcium concentrated outside cells.) Magnesium is the major regulator of the electrical potential on nerve cells. If you are low in magnesium, the electrical charge on the cell is too low and the cell becomes more easily excitable or agitated.

Magnesium deficiency is a symptom found in virtually every single disease and, even in people without significant disease, low magnesium levels are common. On the other hand, some individuals who may have a stronger constitution and tolerate greater stress may tolerate low magnesium levels.

Although magnesium replacement is useful in almost all illnesses, the two illnesses where it has been most successful are fibromyalgia and depression. It is also helpful in diabetes, hypertension, and most other illnesses as well. The problem is magnesium absorption, as well as magnesium deficiency in our diets. The soil in every country in the world except Egypt has been farmed to a point of magnesium depletion. Farmers in the United States know this, and they know that if they don't give their cattle magnesium supplementation, the cattle are likely to die of the "grass staggers," a severe muscular disease leading to death.

There are a number of food items that interfere with magnesium absorption, including high doses of phosphorus. Soda is one of the great contributors to magnesium deficiency, as excess phosphorous interferes tremendously with magnesium absorption, as does high intake of protein and high intake of fat. Soda drinking, high intake of protein, and high intake of fat are all common behaviors in American society. Furthermore, magnesium salts are natural laxatives so that all of them may lead to a more rapid gut transit time. Magnesium needs to travel through the intestinal system slowly, so if the gut transit time is less than twelve hours, one is not likely to absorb the magnesium well.

The best-absorbed oral preparation is **magnesium taurate,** but in my experience, it takes up to one year of oral supplementation to restore intracellular levels to normal. Until a few years ago, I gave most of my patients ten doses of magnesium chloride intravenously over a period of two weeks. This helped to restore the intracellular levels to normal and usually allowed them then to maintain normal levels with oral supplementation. However, one can speed up the process significantly by using Dr. sHEALy's Biogenics® Magnesium Lotion. In four weeks, use of the lotion can accomplish as much as having the ten doses intravenously. It is a lot simpler and easier, and you can do it on your own. There is no known risk to using magnesium unless you have kidney failure.

STRESS IS COMMON AND CANNOT BE TOTALLY AVOIDED, but good nutrition, physical exercise, adequate magnesium, and natural techniques for restoring DHEA are the best ways to handle or minimize stress. In addition, as I will show in a later chapter, relaxation and self-regulation are major antidotes to stress.

3

ANTIDOTES TO STRESS: EXERCISE, HEALTHFUL EATING, AND HEALTHFUL SLEEPING

In his 1884 book *Illustrations of the Influence of the Mind Upon the Body in Health and Disease*,* Dr. Daniel Tuke opened by quoting the great physician John Hunter: "There is not a natural action in the Body, whether involuntary or voluntary, that may not be influenced by the peculiar state of the mind at the time."

That the mind is a powerful influence over the body is hardly news. But Dr. Tuke emphasized the influence of emotions upon every organ in the body. In particular, he emphasized the importance of muscle contraction and muscle relaxation.

---

*This was published in London by J. N. A. Churchill, 11 New Burlington Street, in 1884.

A couple decades after Tuke published his book, Emile Coué, a French pharmacist, began positing that will always yields to imagination. Unfortunately, despite the fact that Coué was credited by European physicians with "curing" more than ten thousand patients with his theory that repeating the phrase "Every day, in every way, I am getting better and better," while invoking the image, would cure an ill person, he was laughed off the stage when he visited the United States.

Then, in 1929, Dr. Edmond Jacobson published his classic work, *Progressive Relaxation* (University of Chicago Press, 1929). Jacobson's ideas were markedly different from Coué's, for Jacobson put his entire emphasis on the principle of teaching relaxation. Jacobson contended that relaxation did not require imagination or willpower or even autosuggestion. Instead, it could be learned, like a skill.

Jacobson would begin by having the patient lie comfortably on his back with arms at the side and legs uncrossed. He often had several patients in the office at once, though in separate rooms, and would walk from room to room instructing the patients to practice specific muscle tension followed by muscle relaxation. Jacobson taught his patients to recognize what muscle tension felt like, and what muscle relaxation felt like. Each group of muscles would be tensed systematically, and in specific order, such as: left biceps, left triceps, left-hand flexors, left-hand extensors, right biceps, right triceps, etc., tensing and relaxing each group of muscles twice and moving slowly down through the body as a whole. Although it seems simple now, Jacobson's methods were revolutionary. He always stressed that muscle tension required effort whereas relaxation did not. Further, he always worked on only one muscle group at a time, emphasizing that the patient should not watch what was happening but instead *feel* what was happening.

Patients were to begin practicing five to fifteen minutes each day.

Gradually they worked up to a total of thirty minutes each day. The improvements in his patients' physical states were clear: Jacobson demonstrated that the knee jerk becomes remarkably diminished during deep relaxation. He measured many physiological activities during deep muscle relaxation, including galvanic skin response (increased during relaxation), gastric secretions, etc. Pulse and blood pressure also were found to decrease during the relaxed state. He noticed 80 percent success in treating colitis, spastic esophagus, chronic insomnia, compulsive neuroses, mild phobias, neurasthenia (chronic fatigue), easy fatigability, anxiety, cardiac neuroses, compulsive tics, depression, Grave's disease (hyperthyroidism), hypochondriasis, generalized spastic paresis, and stuttering and stammering. Although other techniques have been found to be equally useful in alleviating some of the same symptoms, none has been found to be superior to Jacobson's progressive relaxation approach.

AUTOGENIC TRAINING

Beginning his work at almost the same time but not publishing his first book until 1932, J. H. Schultz introduced the concept of **autogenic training**, a self-hypnosis approach. Schultz's goal was to ease and eventually eliminate the dependence a patient felt upon her therapist. The goal was self-regulation. Having noticed that hypnotized subjects experienced feelings of relaxation and heaviness in their extremities, Schultz devised a technique of passive repetition of physiologically oriented statements.

Schultz decreed that the practice should be carried out in a quiet room with low lighting and that the patient should repose in a position that felt most relaxed to her, with all restrictive clothing loosened. If the patient were lying down, Schultz felt the knees should be supported or slightly apart so the heels were not touching. The patient's trunk, shoulders, and head should be in a symmetrical relaxed position. Fingers were to be slightly spread and flexed but should not touch the trunk. The patient was then instructed to concentrate in a goal-directed, focused fashion, essentially an active mental process, although Schultz called it "passive concentration." He instructed patients to use verbal, acoustic, and visual methods of tuning in to various parts of the body.

This sort of therapy was believed by Schultz to combat the physiological alterations induced by stress. In the words of Schultz and his student Wolfgang Luthe, autogenic therapy was "mental manipulations of psychophysiological functions." They supported their statements of success by pointing to research that demonstrated that standard autogenic exercises lead to stabilization or autoregulation of circulation, respiration, and neuromuscular activity. Although most people feel rested and at peace, or tranquil, during the practice of these simple autogenic phrases, an occasional patient has violent emotional outbursts or even flare-ups of symptoms in various organs, which Schultz identified as "brain directed unloading or autogenic discharges." Schultz and Luthe were often working with severely neurotic or psychoneurotic individuals and perhaps sometimes psychotic individuals, and introduced these phrases one at a time.

However, in working with some thirty thousand patients, I have found it perfectly reasonable to introduce all the basic autogenic phrases in the first session, which typically lasts a minimum of ten to fifteen minutes and gradually increases to a twenty-minute practice. Of all the techniques, I have found this one most satisfactory. The phrases are:

My arms and legs are heavy and warm.

My heartbeat is calm and regular.

My breathing is free and easy.

My abdomen is warm.

My forehead is cool.

My mind is quiet and still.

Even with the first practice session, as confirmed in my patients, blood pressure and pulse go down about 10 percent. Just as with progressive relaxation, the knee jerk becomes diminished during autogenic training and patients develop an increased electrical skin resistance, or GSR. Almost all patients benefit within a week or two from practicing this type of mental self-hypnosis or self-regulation therapy, but it takes three to six months for the major benefit of autogenic training to manifest. Schultz always warned that patients should not enter meditation practice until they have mastered the physiological balancing techniques. One usually becomes proficient after, at minimum, six months.

Clinical therapeutic success with autogenic training has been achieved in a great variety of illnesses, including peptic ulcers, hypertension, diabetes, epilepsy, constipation, colitis, spastic colon, nausea, vomiting, and even hemorrhoids. Problems with sexual performance, headaches, various respiratory complaints, gastrointestinal complaints, many cardiac complaints, phobias, anxiety, and insomnia all have been reported to improve with autogenic training. Autogenic training has also been used quite successfully by athletes, as well as various creative artists. Students often improve academically. In Germany, a number of autogenic training sessions have been carried out under the auspices of various business organizations such as the Chamber of Commerce to increase health and efficiency and decrease absenteeism, as well as to decrease errors and accidents, improve interpersonal relationships, and lessen stress overall. Of the 2,600 references in *Autogenic Training,* vol. 1 (Grune and Stratton, New York, 1969), less than 10 percent are in English and most of them came from Japan. America has yet to fully catch on to this relaxation technique.

I have a few autogenic resources that have proven useful to some, including my tape, *Basic Schultz.* A twelve-minute autogenic exercise, this tape has been used by many hundreds of individuals, resulting in great benefit. (In fact, one doctoral student did his doctoral dissertation using this in patients with fibromyalgia and had remarkably good success.) It has also been of great use to individuals with depression and anxiety.

My book *90 Days to Stress-Free Living* presents the wide variety of stress-reducing techniques that I have found most effective in my patients. In it, you will find a more lengthy discussion of relaxation techniques, including practices for physical, mental, emotional, and spiritual balancing. It is important to have a wide variety of techniques at hand in order to learn how to balance or control physical sensation, and the book provides a number of exercises for balancing emotions, for negotiating unfinished emotional business, and, finally, for spiritual attunement.

PHOTOSTIMULATION

Over the course of my career, I have worked with over thirty thousand people who were suffering from various chronic illnesses. Many of these patients used **photostimulation** as an adjunct for deep relaxation. Also known as "light therapy," photostimulation aids in relaxation by exposing the patient to doses of light. Virtually all people suffering from depression experience a degree of agitation or anxiety. Photostimulation is particularly helpful in these cases, reducing stress and helping individuals relax without having to think about it, without having to do any of the guided imagery or other exercises outlined above.

The **Shealy RelaxMate II**™ provides photostimulation at a safe frequency of 1 to 7 cycles/second and is optimally relaxing. It has been known since the discovery of the electroencephalogram in the 1920s that the brain "follows" the frequency of flashing lights. And deep relaxation occurs at these lower frequency rates. It also allows the individual to choose between pure blue, pure red, or a mixture of blue and red colors for optimizing their personal sense of relaxation. For those who have trouble relaxing, for those who have trouble with the mind wandering, and for those who do not wish to "work" for relaxation, the Shealy RelaxMate II™ offers the best-known technique. Ninety percent of my patients report themselves in a deep state of relaxation within ten minutes of applying the RelaxMate II™. Once they have selected the frequency and the color preference, all they have to do is put on a pair of glasses that look much like sunglasses and close their eyes. We recommend it be used a minimum of twenty minutes a day up to an hour a day. It can be used at any time and at bedtime (leave the timer on for one hour and fall asleep in the relaxed state).

BIOFEEDBACK TRAINING

In the early 1970s, Dr. Elmer Green introduced the concept of **biofeedback.** A technique that encourages patients to use signals from their own bodies to relax themselves, biofeedback is literally a "feeding back" of information from your body *about* your body. This treatment is widely used by physical therapists who aid patients in recovery from illnesses like strokes, which have paralyzed muscles in various parts of the body. Others use biofeedback to help patients learn to relax. Biofeedback has been discovered useful in a wide variety of stress illnesses, ranging from migraine headaches to tension headaches to hypertension. It has also been of great use in managing various types of chronic pain.

The simplest and easiest biofeedback technique to learn is **temperature control.** By applying even a simple fifty-cent thermometer taped to the index finger, one can learn to raise one's temperature from the "normal" skin temperature of 85 to 90 degrees up to at least 96 degrees. This self-control achieves optimal reduction of the body's stress reaction. Just feeling the pulse of the heartbeat in the fingertip or imagining the sun beaming its rays upon the fingers, individuals can learn to control their reaction to stress. With this technique, individuals are learning control of their sympathetic autonomic, or "automatic," nervous system, which is at the core of our overreactions to stress.

PHYSICAL EXERCISE

Genetic influences on an individual's aging process have been highly overrated. Much more important than predisposition are an individual's levels of alcohol consumption and stress, his diet, and the amount of physical exercise he engages in.[27] In fact, physical exercise may be the single most important determinant of health. Those who choose not to be couch potatoes already have a positive attitude and, generally, greater motivation to be healthy. Furthermore, people who exercise regularly tend to eat better than those who don't, and those who take up exercise in midlife are likely to simultaneously improve their eating habits.

Until around midcentury, the majority of people were reasonably active in their everyday lives—simple chores required labor. However, beginning around 1940, when labor-saving appliances such as washing machines began appearing in American homes, the physical demands of the typical day decreased. Before my mother got her first washing machine in the 1940s, she boiled clothes in a large iron pot in the backyard. She had to stir the clothes, do much physical activity to get them clean, then wring them out by hand.

But, of course, nothing has decreased the physical activity of the average American more than the arrival of a remarkably addictive appliance: the television. With average people spending twenty-five- to forty-five-plus hours per week watching the "boob tube," physical activity has hit an all-time low, perhaps lower than at any time in the entire evolution of humanity. With hundreds of physiological and longevity studies now proving unequivocally that physical exercise is one of the greatest determinants of health, state of the body, and mind, as well as longevity, inactivity should not be an option.

Consider the following facts: Long-term endurance training significantly improves the autonomic nervous system's control of the heart. It increases the vegetative (read: *healing*) activity and decreases sympathetic (read: *stress*) activity. The **sympathetic nervous system** is the fight-or-flight "adrenaline" mechanism. The **parasympathetic nervous system** is the opposite—it regulates metabolism, digestion, etc. It has been shown that *decreased* parasympathetic activity is associated with physiological aging. Interestingly, in general, and obviously there are exceptions, women tend to have greater parasympathetic activity and men have greater sympathetic activity throughout life. This factor alone may be the major difference in longevity between men and women.[28]

Physical fitness and obesity are totally and unequivocally inversely related. It is almost impossible to study the effects of physical activity without also incorporating the concepts and adverse effects of obesity.

Fitness is generally assessed using a treadmill stress test; but true fitness is associated with decreased mortality from *all causes*, not just cardiovascular disease. Also, increased obesity is associated with increased mortality from *all causes*, among these cardiovascular disease.[29]

Physical exercise in "older" adults has been shown to significantly improve longevity.[30] In fact, one study found that "no single segment of our society can benefit more from regularly performed exercise and improved diet than elderly adults."[31] In addition, most studies have demonstrated a strong association between moderately vigorous and vigorous exercise and lower instances of coronary heart disease in people from ages thirty-five to the mid-sixties.[32] Other studies have demonstrated an excellent consensus showing decreased morbidity and mortality from coronary artery disease, stroke and cardiovascular disease, and cancer correlating with both physical fitness as well as physical activity. And there is a gradient—that is, the greater the fitness and the greater the physical exercise, the stronger the health benefits.[33] In fact, in addition to cardiovascular fitness, a number of studies show that physical exercise decreases arthritis. (In general, no matter how significant the arthritis, physical exercise, even when there is pain, is far healthier for individuals than inactivity.[34])

One of the most important signs of aging is a decrease in

the growth hormone the body produces. Physical exercise *induces* growth-hormone response. Specifically, resistance training and other forms of moderate to intense physical activity all induce this positive response (the amount of the response is associated with intensity, duration, frequency, and mode of endurance exercise).

In order to reap the benefits of physical activity, it must be at least mildly rigorous, or "moderate." Light physical activities are *not* associated with reduced mortality rates. Although nonvigorous exercise has many benefits on health in general, it does not increase longevity, whereas vigorous activity strongly increases longevity.[35] A good example of moderate activity is a three-to-four-mile walk each day, the sort of activity that is strongly associated with increased longevity. But an even greater benefit can be drawn from more vigorous activity.[36] (The benefits hardly stop at the physiological level; memory, too, is improved by physical exercise.[37])

Inactivity can promote a variety of potentially serious blood abnormalities such as lower blood plasma volume (allowing blood to sludge), higher hematocrit (concentration of hemoglobin), higher plasma fibrinogen (easier clotting), elevated blood viscosity (easier clotting), increased platelet aggregability (greater clotting), and diminished fibrinolysis (greater clotting). In other words, inactivity greatly increases the potential for the "sludging" of blood and clots, especially in the heart and brain.[38] Inactivity is also associated with marked and debilitating psychiatric conditions ranging from panic disorder, hypochondriasis, depression, and multiple phobias.[39]

It has been unequivocally proven that a sedentary lifestyle leads to decreased strength, flexibility of muscles, and flexibility of joints; and, especially in the flexibility of the cardiovascular system, it appears that a minimum ideal is one hour of formal exercise per day at all ages, at least from about age five.[40] Unfortunately only 22 percent of Americans are "regularly active." This means, of course, that 78 percent are inactive![41] The good news is that previously sedentary, reasonably healthy adults who enter a structured exercise program of increased physical activity achieve significant improvements in reduction of blood pressure, loss of body fat and, of course, overall health and longevity![42]

One form of physical exercise that is rarely assessed in longevity studies is sexual activity. There are a number of studies suggesting that sexual activity is associated with well-being and longevity. This may come not only from the physical exercise involved but also the improved neurochemistry associated with love and nurturing.[43]

The bottom line is that our levels of physical activity determine how we age: Individuals with better health habits not only survive longer, but the disabilities associated with aging are also postponed.[44]

WHAT KIND OF EXERCISE?

What type of exercise should you do? Well, halitosis is better than no breath at all, and any activity is better than no activity. The time of day when you exercise is also important: There is excellent evidence that exercise early in the morning—before breakfast—has greater benefit on caloric expenditures throughout the day than exercise at the end of the day. Personally, I prefer to get up early and exercise before breakfast. My own exercise program consists of a minimum of four hours per week on a Health Rider® with fifty pounds of weight on it, 100 sit-ups and 100 back-ups each day on a Roman chair, and walking thirty to sixty minutes every day, as well as a minimum of twenty minutes of yoga daily.

From a cardiovascular point of view, it is a question of **aerobic points**. Adequate (*optimal*) physical exercise means getting forty-five to sixty aerobics points per week. Ideally, optimal health requires a minimum of four and a maximum of six days of exercise per week. Thus, I encourage you to plan for ten to fifteen aerobics points each exercise period. It will take at least three months to reach this exercise intensity and, if you are in poor shape initially, it may take six months.

Which of the following are you *willing to develop*?

Walking	4 miles in 60 min. = 11 points
	5 miles in 75 min. = 14 points
Jogging	3 miles in 36 min. = 11 points
	4 miles in 48 min. = 15 points
	3 miles in 30 min. = 14 points
Jogging on a Trampoline	120 steps/min. = 1 point/4 min.
	180 steps/min. = 1 point/3 min.
	240 steps/min. = 1 point/2 min.
Stationary Bike	at 35 mph = 1 point/3 min.
Racquetball	10 points/60 min.

(If you prefer swimming or some other sport, check one of Dr. Kenneth Cooper's many books on aerobic exercise.[45])

In addition to cardiovascular physical exercise, you need **limbering**. This allows muscles, joints, and tendons to remain optimally flexible. Optimal flexibility helps prevent the stiffness and impaired mobility so common in the elderly. I strongly recommend the following limbering exercises. Remember that these should be comfortable and fun. Start with what you can do easily and build gradually. (See Figures 3.1–3.5.)

Limbering (Flexibility) Exercises

Twirling

With the arms stretched out at shoulder height, turn clockwise (toward the right). Start by doing not more than 2 or 3 twirls and build up gradually over a period of 2 or 3 weeks to 21 twirls a day.

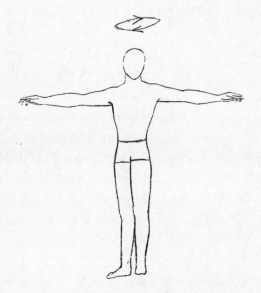

Figure 3.1 Twirling

Head and Leg Raises

Lying flat on your back on a firm surface with your hands beside your buttocks, take a deep breath in and, as you breathe out, raise your legs straight up into the air. At the same time, raise your head up as if you were going to touch your head to your knees. Knees are kept straight. Then, as legs and head are lowered to the floor, take another deep breath. Again, start off with 2 or 3 exercises and build up over a period of 2 or 3 weeks to a total of 21.

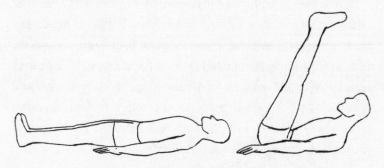

Figure 3.2 HEAD AND LEG RAISES

Back Arches

On a carpeted floor, keep your body erect while kneeling. Bend your head forward onto your chest and take a deep breath. As you breathe out, bend your head back as far as it will go, keeping your thighs straight up, arching your head and back maximally. You may put your hands behind the lower part of your buttocks to give additional stability. Start with 2 or 3 repetitions and build to 21.

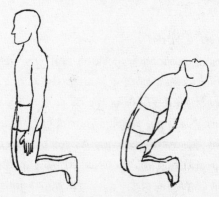

Figure 3.3 BACK ARCHES

The Table

While sitting with your legs straight out in front, put your palms flat on the floor directly beside your buttocks. Bend your head forward as you breathe out and raise your knees up into the air to make your thighs parallel with the floor, keeping your calves perpendicular to the floor. At the same time, arch your head and neck backward. This makes your body, from the shoulders down to the knees, parallel with the floor and gives the appearance of your body being a table. Start with 2 repetitions and build to 21.

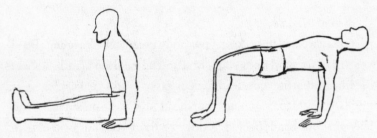

Figure 3.4 THE TABLE

Modified Cobra

Put yourself facedown in position as if you were doing push-ups, with your toes supporting your body at one end and your palms flat down on the floor at the other end. Extend your head back as far as it will go, arching your upper back, keeping your knees straight. Take a deep breath. As you breathe out, bend your head forward and bring your buttocks straight up into the air, keeping your knees straight. Start with 2 repetitions and build to 21.

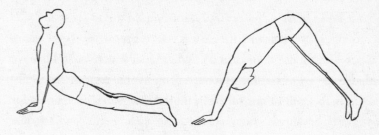

Figure 3.5 MODIFIED COBRA

Sit-ups

In addition, sit-ups with your knees bent are excellent for abdominal strengthening: very important in preventing back injuries.

If you walk, jog, or use a trampoline, add Heavy Hands® or a type of dumbbell that can add great extra exercise to your upper body and heart. You can start with one pound in each hand and build up to 10. Even simple dumbbells can be used.

YOU CANNOT AFFORD A SEDENTARY LIFESTYLE. IF YOU can commit to an active physical lifestyle for at least three months, chances are that your health and mood will improve significantly and, ideally, you will be motivated to continue this for the rest of a much longer and healthier life.

Alternative Exercises

If you don't want to start with aerobic activity or the exercises that I have indicated here, there is a pattern called "The Daily Dozen Exercises" from Edgar Cayce's writings. (See Appendix A.)

These twelve exercises offer another significant pattern to keep your body flexible. Jeffrey Furst introduced me to these in 1972, and indeed, this may be the easiest way for most people to begin. Start with whatever you can do, and gradually increase it. I believe that if you will do twenty-one repetitions of each of the Daily Dozen, this will be one of the healthiest things that you can do for yourself, because it would include adequate limbering and, to some extent, cardiovascular strengthening exercise. Indeed, if you would just do the "Jangles" two or three minutes every waking hour, that in itself would be a remarkably beneficial exercise program.

THE PARADOX OF EXTREMES: NUTRITION AND DIETS

Nutrition is perhaps the most disputed aspect of health. Consider these diet extremes, and then look at my most recommended nutritional plan.

THE RICE DIET

Pioneered at Duke University by Dr. Walter Kempner, the Rice Diet[46] virtually cures many diabetics, severe hypertensives, and the obese. The diet consists of all you can eat of:

White rice
Canned sweetened fruit
One simple daily vitamin containing RDA
If you're not obese or diabetic, all the white sugar you want!

Contents: Protein 20 grams
Fat 0
Carbohydrates unlimited, simple and starch
Sodium 100 mg./day

The rice diet is an extreme and must be done under careful medical supervision. But for the massively obese or those whose blood pressure is dangerously high, it may be considered. It is by far the most difficult of all the diets I have reviewed.

THE ATKINS DIET

Excellent for weight loss in about 80 percent of people, the Atkins Diet[47] lowers cholesterol. It consists of:

Unlimited meat, cheese, eggs, low-starch vegetables
No grains or alcohol
Contents: Protein, 75 to 150+ grams
Fat, 250+ grams
Carbohydrate, 10 to 30 grams

The major problem with the Atkins Diet is the need to assure a high intake of water. About 5 percent of individuals become nauseated and do not tolerate the Atkins Diet. About 10 percent do not lose weight.

THE DIFFERENCE IN THESE TWO EXTREMES IS THE COMbination of fat and carbohydrates: no fat in the Rice Diet and almost unlimited fat with minimal carbohydrates in the Atkins Diet. For many people, the combination of fat and carbohydrates is nearly toxic and is the obesity-producing combination. When you eat carbohydrates, you tend to store them as fat. Thus on a high-carbohydrate diet, fat is the culprit. When you do not have adequate carbohydrates for energy needs, you *burn* fat and do not store it. The Atkins Diet is monotonous but works well for weight control and keeping cholesterol optimal in many people. You must drink adequate water (about two quarts daily) and take an excellent multivitamin when you are on this diet.

Other excellent and somewhat more tasty diets are:

MACROBIOTIC

Mainly fish (boiled, poached, baked)
Brown rice
Steamed vegetables
Seaweed seasonings
Contents: Protein, approximately 50 grams
Carbohydrate, moderate
Fat, less than 20 grams

It is good for weight control and immune enhancement. For individuals with cancer, allergies, and immune weakness, this is an excellent diet.

THE METABOLIC TYPING DIET[48]

Pioneered by Dr. George Watson, this diet provides a Western assessment very similar to Ayurvedic medicine. Watson divides people into:

Fast oxidizers—who need lots of protein and fat

Slow oxidizers—who are more satisfied with high carbohydrate diets, moderate protein and low fat

Mixed—the small percentage of people who appear to be
true omnivores

In Ayurvedic terms:

Fast oxidizers = Pita

Slow Oxidizers = Kaptha

Mixed = Vata

THE SHEALY COMMONSENSE DIET

In general, if you maintain your ideal weight, I think a *wide variety* of real food is your best bet. This is compatible with Cayce's recommendations, and it is my major recommendation!

Meats of all kinds—beef, pork, chicken, turkey, fish, etc.,
4 to 16 oz./day

Fresh vegetables—as many raw as possible. Minimize
starchy vegetables, especially Irish potatoes.

Sweet potatoes are *excellent* if you do not add sugar.

Cheese, yogurt, buttermilk—unlimited

Brown rice—as desired

Oatmeal and other whole-grain cereals (NOT boxed
  dry cereals)

Truly 100 percent whole-grain breads (2–3 slices daily)

Eggs, 1 to 3 daily

Dry-roasted peanuts and *old-fashioned* peanut butter
  (Smuckers® is excellent): 1 to 4 tablespoons daily

Almonds, pecans, walnuts, cashews, sunflower seeds,
    etc.—2 to 3 oz. daily (depending on total calories
    needed to maintain normal weight)

Dried legumes cooked—up to 1 cup daily

Fresh fruits—unlimited

VEGAN

The "pure" vegetarian represents less than 1 percent of Americans, and even lacto-ovo vegetarians account for a total of only 4 percent of Americans. I have observed scores of vegetarians who are borderline unhealthy at best and often are far less healthy than heavy meat eaters. Two critical factors seem important:

1. **Vegetable protein is not as easily digestible.** Furthermore, it is totally lacking in taurine, one of the most important amino acids. Every vegan I have tested is deficient in one to several essential amino acids.

2. **There is no vitamin B_{12} in vegetables;** only eggs, milk products, and various fresh foods contain B_{12}. Eventually all pure vegans are likely to become B_{12} deficient.

There is NO scientific evidence that meat is harmful to health. On the contrary, it is nearly essential for optimal health. Fish is especially good!

Finally, among Seventh-Day Adventists, pure vegetarian females have an increased risk of death from heart disease. This is particularly striking since Seventh-Day Adventists, in general, have increased longevity largely because of no smoking, no alcohol, and strong faith.

METABOLIC SYNDROME, OR SYNDROME X

With diet, it is important to consider how your body responds to and processes carbohydrates. At least 25 percent of normal, otherwise healthy, nonobese individuals have a genetic predisposition to producing excessive amounts of insulin when carbohydrates are eaten. About 50 percent of individuals seem to tolerate carbohydrates reasonably well, and 25 percent of individuals, especially the slow oxidizers, tolerate carbohydrates very well indeed, with low production of insulin.

The 25 percent of healthy nonobese individuals who overrespond to carbohydrates with an excess insulin reaction are prone to hypoglycemia and eventually develop mature-onset diabetes, despite their lack of obesity; this leads to insulin resistance and many negative physiological responses, a group of symptoms commonly called **Syndrome X**. Individuals with Syndrome X are at increased risk for diabetes, heart disease, hypertension, stroke, polycystic ovary syndrome, breast cancer, elevated serum uric acid, elevated triglycerides, low HDL, elevated LDL, rheumatoid arthritis, and eventually obesity. These individuals tend to store fat in the abdominal area.

SYMPTOMS AND SIGNS OF SYNDROME X

Hunger soon after eating

Irritability an hour or two after eating

Frequent fatigue

More than 10 pounds overweight

Mental sluggishness

High blood pressure

High blood triglycerides

High cholesterol

High fasting blood sugar

Low blood sugar two to three hours after eating

Insulin resistance essentially develops from a combination of genetic, environmental, and dietary influences. In Syndrome X, there is **hyperinsulinemia**. The result is poor glucose regulation, increased LDL, increased triglycerides, increased abdominal obesity, hypertension, increased uric acid, and decreased HDL leading to the diseases already identified. One of the relatively early signs of Syndrome X is slight damage to the kidneys from metabolic excess, which allows the kidneys to "leak" serum protein. Eventually this can lead to kidney damage, hypertension, and even kidney failure.

Another element of diet to keep an eye on is antioxidant levels. Low levels of many antioxidants are associated with hypertension. For instance, lower levels of vitamin A (preferably beta-carotene) and vitamin C are associated with 43 percent and 18 percent higher odds of hypertension, respectively. With deficiencies of vitamins A and E, the effect is both **systolic** and **diastolic,** whereas with vitamin-C deficiency it is primarily associated with diastolic blood pressure elevation.[49] Be certain that your diet includes sufficient levels of important antioxidants, especially if you are on one of the "extreme" diets outlined above. Raw fruits such as blueberries, grapes, and raspberries and cooked vegetables such as broccoli are the best sources of antioxidants.

For most individuals, I recommend a good multivitamin containing a least 25 mg. of B complex, 25,000 units of beta-carotene, and 400 units of vitamin E. Then you also need at least 1,000 mg. of calcium, especially calcium citrate; 1,000 units of vitamin D, and magnesium, best obtained by using magnesium lotion. Magnesium is notoriously erratic in intestinal absorption.

When it comes to fats, coconut oil is among the most interesting. In general, it is one of the few fats that I recommend, in addition to olive oil and butter, and it has health benefits at least equal to those of olive oil. It is a good occasional oil to use, but it is much more expensive than either olive oil or butter, and it does taste like coconut! You also need each day at least a couple of grams of the essential Omega-3 fatty acids found in a good fish oil. I much prefer capsules of these.

TRACE ELEMENTS

There are over 29,000 published medical research papers dealing with **trace elements** in the Archives of the National Library of Medicine. The research here is substantial and somewhat overwhelming. For instance, illnesses associated with low levels of zinc include: childhood hyperactivity, tuberculosis, rheumatoid arthritis, many cancers, multiple sclerosis, arthritis, goiter, Down's syndrome, mental retardation, Alzheimer's, hepatic fibrosis, liver disease, liver cancer, gallstones, hepatitis, cirrhosis, breast cancer, and a weak immune system.[50]

A wide variety of trace elements—including bismuth, cesium, cobalt, copper, manganese, rubidium, zinc, and magnesium—are all involved in one way or another with coronary artery disease.[51]

In addition to these trace elements, folic acid and vitamin B_{12} are important supplements because of the increasing level of **homocysteine** that occurs with age. Homocysteine is an independent predictor of hypertension. Adjusting for all the cardiovascular risk factors, an elevation of homocysteine above the midrange of so-called normal is associated with increases in both diastolic and systolic blood pressure in both men and women. Women are at three times greater risk of having hypertension between the highest and lowest levels of homocysteine, whereas men have only a twofold increase between the highest and lowest levels. Another article suggests that having an elevated level of homocysteine is a risk factor for estrogen-induced hormonal cancer.[52] In other words, you really want to be in the lowest range of homocysteine, and this can be accomplished in almost everyone by taking adequate amounts of folic acid plus vitamin B_{12}. **A minimum of 5 mg. of folic acid (and in some individuals, 100 mg.) and 1,000 mcg. daily of vitamin B_{12} should be taken.** The latter may be taken sublingually.[53]

Tribulus terrestris, a Chinese herb, has been found to reduce **angina pectoris** by 82.3 percent in 406 cases. In addition to its potential effect in increasing testosterone and helping alleviate erectile dysfunction, *tribulus terrestris* dilates coronary arteries and improves coronary circulation. It appears to have no adverse effects on the blood system, the liver, or the kidneys, and there are no known side effects. The Chinese consider it "one of the ideal medications to treat angina pectoris."[54]

SLEEP

One of the most neglected factors in health and longevity is sleep, both in terms of the length of sleep and its quality. In the late 1700s, the average American got ten hours of sleep. Today the average is about five hours. The effect of such incredibly shortened sleep hours is remarkably complex and often devastating. Human performance is markedly dependent upon good-quality sleep, and nowhere is this problem of sleep inadequacy more flagrantly ignored than among the leaders of American industry. As equipment and systems increase in complexity and reliability, rates of human error have not kept pace—indeed, cannot keep pace—without acknowledging the necessity of adequate sleep. Long-haul truckers work a fifteen-hour day.[55] Medical interns and physicians work thirty-six-hour shifts. The majority of serious accidents occur at night. In only 200 years, a society that had been dependent upon the cycles of light and dark began ignoring hundreds of thousands of years of evolutionary adaptability. Some argue that the Industrial Revolution separated us from major natural cycles, including our natural tendency to sleep when it gets dark and get up when it gets light.

Circadian rhythm, that physiological response to the roughly twenty-four-hour daylight cycle, has been shown unequivocally to affect a wide variety of functions ranging from body temperature to the levels of most of our hormones. Dr. Martin Moore-Ede has demonstrated that it is possible for industry not only to address these issues but also to improve productivity quite strikingly.[56]

The **electroencephalogram (EEG)** is one good way to look at how we appear in our normal, bright-eyed, bushy-tailed, alert state. The EEG of an alert person produces electrical waves at a frequency of 13 to 35 cycles per second. As we settle into a state of relaxation, brain waves slow to between 8 and 12 cycles per second, called the **alpha range**. Those who practice relaxation for long periods of time can maintain this level. As we slow down further, the brain begins to produce **theta waves** at 3 to 7 cycles per second. This is the stage often associated with spontaneous imagery and creativity. We then slip into the deepest stage of sleep, **delta**, at a rhythm of 0.5 to 2 cycles per second. Throughout the rest of the night, we vary significantly in the brain wave frequency and, just as during our daylight hours, we then have 90-minute cycles. Four to five times every night, and in some individuals many more, we dream. During this time, the brain-wave activity goes back into frequencies associated with alertness, such as a **beta stage**, and our eyes start moving rapidly from side to side. This is called **REM**, or rapid-eye-movement sleep. Most people who have had a good night's sleep wake up slowly and are wide awake, but if you happen to wake up from the deepest stages of delta, you are likely to feel groggy and disoriented. And, if you wake up immediately after a dream, you are likely to be the most bright eyed of all.

In the majority of individuals there is an intrinsic tendency to become drowsy in the early afternoon, and it occurs whether or not you are hungry and whether or not you eat lunch. This biological clock is controlled from a small area in the brain called the suprachiasmatic nucleus (SCN). It receives tremendous input from the eyes about light and dark. Disturbances in this biological clock can result in severe problems, such as falling asleep too easily (as in the case of narcoleptics, who have great difficulty staying awake).

Interestingly, individuals who are deprived of all aspects of daylight and become research subjects in specialized sleep labs change their sleep patterns drastically. In one study some individuals would adopt a thirty-six-hour day and occasionally even up to a fifty-hour day. Interestingly, they still ate only three meals during their waking time, but their sleep periods increased to fifteen or even twenty or more hours.[57] This study indicates that even in such situations, individuals sleep a full third of the time. More important, individuals who are accustomed to going to sleep at a specific hour develop a pattern, and reasonably healthy individuals tend to wake up after specific periods of sleep so that going to bed later than average rarely is associated with a longer sleep cycle. Nowhere is this more obvious than in international travel. Individuals vary considerably in how long it takes them to adjust to time-zone changes. Westward travel is generally much easier for people than travel toward the east. It takes individuals flying westward anywhere from two to eight days to accommodate to a six-hour time-zone change, whereas if they fly eastward it takes four to eighteen days to adjust to the same six-hour change. It is the suprachiasmatic nucleus, or SCN, biological clock that determines our response to light in general. (Tip for jeg-lagged travelers: Sometimes darkening the eyes as completely as possible helps to reset the biological time clock.)

For most individuals, peak alertness during the day occurs when they have slept *between eight and nine hours at night*. Alertness is a complex mechanism that is related to: sense of danger, interest, or opportunity; muscle activity; time of day on the circadian cycle; one's sleep reserves; total nutrition; environmental light; environmental temperature; environmental sound; and environmental aroma or smell.

Bright lights markedly reduce drowsiness. Cool, dry air makes one much more alert, as does a cold shower, and these are associated with appropriate stimulation of the sympathetic nervous system. Irregular and variable sound tends to keep us awake and arouse the sympathetic nervous system, whereas a rather monotonous sound lulls one into sleep.

Studies at the University of Chicago have demonstrated that deeper, slow-wave sleep that occurs about 20 percent of the time in young individuals decreases to less than 5 percent for those over age thirty-five, with growth-hormone secretion decreasing by about 75 percent. The average amount of sleep decreases by almost one half hour every decade after age fifty. REM sleep or dream sleep also decreases by about 50 percent after age fifty.[58]

So how do we remedy this? One of the greatest problems in today's society is the use of various and sundry psychotropic drugs.[59] For many years 25 to 50 mg. of amitriptyline at bedtime was used to enhance sleep. The result was a large decrease in REM time. Further, at least 25 percent of the people taking amitriptyline have significant adverse effects, which is true of most of the antidepressants. Indeed, none of the antidepressants enhances the quality of sleep. Other sleep concerns include:

- Sleep deprivation: A deprivation of only forty-eight hours leads to poor production of DNA, significantly decreasing one's immune health and longevity![60]

- Sleep apnea: This is another major problem of inadequate sleep or sleep interference. The common concept that sleep patterns change after a warm bath has actually been studied. Individuals who take a warm bath at bedtime had significant increases in sleepiness, slow-wave sleep, and deep sleep, although REM sleep was reduced, especially in the first REM sleep.[61]

- Relatively minor changes in sleep: These small changes do have an effect, and sleep deprivation of as little as two hours has clear negative effects on alertness. Six hours of sleep is too short for optimal alertness in the vast majority of people.[62]

- Subliminal arousal: It has also been demonstrated that individuals who are subliminally aroused, such as those who sleep near an airport where they accommodate and don't wake up totally when planes fly, have decreased quality of sleep and adverse health effects.

- Fibromyalgia and chronic fatigue syndrome: Perhaps no chronic diseases are more specifically related to poor sleep than fibromyalgia and chronic fatigue syndrome.[63] In both of these situations, decreases occur in growth hormone, DHEA, melatonin, and a wide number of neurohormones.

- Magnesium levels: As I emphasized in the section on magnesium in chapter 2, and as you might expect, magnesium is very much involved in sleep regulation, as so many chemicals are dependent upon adequate magnesium presence in the body. DHEA deficiencies, as just one example, lead to insomnia.

MELATONIN

Melatonin is considered a major hormone for regulating sleep.[64] A free-radical scavenger, melatonin also has antioxidant properties. It improves rapid-eye movement sleep and helps to restore growth-hormone secretion.[65] Melatonin may induce sleep when the homeostatic mechanism is insufficient and may help induce phase shifts in the circadian clock. Other important facts about melatonin to consider include:

- Individuals who normally sleep longer periods, greater than nine hours, have increased cortisol levels, lower body temperature, and higher plasma melatonin levels. Indeed, the normal increase in cortisol, which occurs usually as we wake up, occurs about 2.5 hours later in long sleepers than in short sleepers.[66] In primary insomnia, nocturnal melatonin production is significantly diminished.

- Sleep is strikingly related to the amount and time of **tryptophan** administration. Midmorning administration of a high-protein diet or of tryptophan delays REM sleep latency (duration of sleep from sleep onset to the onset of the first REM sleep period), whereas tryptophan at bedtime shortens sleep latency.[67] It is important to know that tryptophan is converted into serotonin and serotonin into melatonin.

- Sleep times are significantly increased by melatonin given at bedtime. Melatonin secretion is significantly reduced by a late-evening carbohydrate-rich meal, whereas a carbohydrate-rich meal in the morning does not significantly increase melatonin production.[68]

- One hundred mg. of pyridoxine at bedtime does not enhance melatonin secretion.[69]
- Melatonin appears to be effective in the treatment of tardive dyskinesia but actually may aggravate the tremor in Parkinsonism.[70]

For some individuals 1 mg. of melotonin is sufficient. Others require at least 21 mg. Even at low doses of 3 mg., some individuals are left feeling hung over and groggy, whereas others at 21 mg. wake up bright eyed and alert! Certainly you should start by trying 3 mg. It should work the first night. If it does not, gradually add another 3 mg. each night until you either sleep soundly or do not awaken bright eyed and alert!

TREATMENT OF INSOMNIA

In my experience, the very best approach to insomnia is stress reduction. The second-best approach is the use of the **Liss TENS™, Shealy Series,** device transcranially, across the temples or forehead to the back of the head, for forty to sixty minutes in the morning, beginning anytime after 6 A.M. and finishing no later than 1 P.M. The Liss stimulator is remarkably safe—it can be used by anyone who does not have an implanted electronic medical device such as a pacemaker. It puts out only 1 to 4 milliamps of current at 15,000 pulses per second, modified 500 and 15 times per second. It is so safe you could drive your car while wearing it—although I do not recommend that, as it might be distracting! It does require a prescription. The Liss stimulator helps reset the total serotonin circadian rhythm and raises beta endorphins, the natural narcotics that make you feel good, safely.

Other healthy approaches to treating insomnia include:

- taking a warm bath two to three hours before bedtime and even up to bedtime.
- taking Tryptophan, 1 to 4 grams, at bedtime. Tryptophan is an essential amino acid and is the building block for serotonin and melatonin. Happily, tryptophan is available over the counter. But note that one must take at least 25 to 100 mg. of vitamin B complex to make this work well. Other adjuncts that may enhance the effect of tryptophan are lithium orotate, up to 45 mg., adequate magnesium intake (particularly keeping one's magnesium level up through the use of something like Biogenics® Magnesium Lotion), 3 to 4 grams of taurine at bedtime, and from 1 to 21 mg. of melatonin at bedtime. Individuals have to explore each of these modalities for themselves, because everyone's body reacts differently, and it is possible that one treatment will work and another will not.
- Probably the best adjunct to sleep that was ever devised is **gamma hydroxybutyrate**, but unfortunately the federal government has made that a very restricted drug. In fact, it was banned for some years but has recently been approved only for treatment of narcolepsy. Of course, once it's on the market, you might, if you are desperate, find

a physician who would prescribe it. It does more than any other known drug to improve the quality and depth of sleep.

Now that I have discussed stress, the major contributor to all illness, it is time to consider some of the most common health problems, specifically depression—perhaps the most common illness in the world.

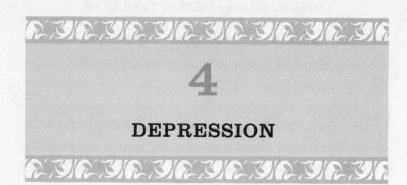

4

DEPRESSION

When Caroline Myss and I wrote *The Creation of Health*, I mentioned that the most "popular" way to die is from heart disease. Why is it so "popular"? Because so many people are carrying around unresolved anger and depression—the emotional issues that create the foundations for disease.

Depression is, in my opinion, the most common illness in the world. Moreover, it appears to be an underlying component of a remarkable number of other illnesses. Depression—specifically chronic depression—not only takes an emotional toll on an individual; it also essentially weakens the immune system and thus leads to multiple disturbances in the entire metabolic control system. Anxiety, anger, and depression strikingly alter the pituitary gland with its output of all the major stimulating hormones for the other endocrine organs, most particularly the thyroid and the adrenals, so that in general there tends to be a disturbance in the normal endocrine output rhythm, particularly of cortisol.

Although psychologists and psychiatrists have devised many categories for depression, in general it seems to me that there is either a fairly pure depression or anxiety with depression. In many people who have an extreme agitated anxiety, it is the underlying depressive aspect that causes the reaction of anxiety itself.

Both anxiety and depression affect the functioning of the pituitary gland, which orchestrates the output of all the major stimulating hormones for other endocrine organs—most particularly the thyroid and the adrenals. So, when a person is depressed or suffering from anxiety, in general there tends to be a disturbance in the normal endocrine output rhythm, particularly of cortisol.

For example, when a healthy person goes to sleep, normally his stress level is significantly reduced, and his cortisol levels go down. When that person awakens and begins participating in the normal activities of the day, cortisol levels begin to rise, usually peaking around 4 P.M. When individuals are depressed, this mechanism is disturbed: The adrenal glands continue to produce a late-afternoon level of cortisol throughout the night, so the next day begins with a higher than normal level of cortisol. Eventually, the total twenty-four-hour production of the hormone is increased. Often accompanied by changes in adrenalin levels, this leads to a fundamental change in the body's basic reaction to stress. Physiologically, it is as if the individual is under significant stress twenty-four hours a day! The threshold for new stress of any kind is then lowered, since there is already an active ongoing biochemical stress reaction.

EYSENCK'S PERSONALITY TYPES

Perhaps one of the most interesting studies of this phenomenon was completed by Hans Eysenck working with a colleague in Germany.[71] Essentially, Eysenck categorized individuals into four basic lifestyle personalities:

Type I individuals tend to have a lifelong pattern of hopelessness. These individuals seem to have had a feeling of abandonment in childhood, and they always want love and nurturing from someone who is not capable of, or interested in, returning that love. Therefore, they often choose an abusive spouse or crave a relationship with someone with whom it is not possible. These Type I individuals have an average life expectancy *35 years less* than certain other types. Incredibly, Eysenck found that 75 percent of adult individuals who die of cancer have a Type I personality, as do 15 percent of adults who die of heart disease.

Type II individuals have a lifelong pattern of severe blame or anger. They feel abused. They often pick fights or constantly act as if they want to pick a fight. *Seventy-five percent* of adults who die of heart disease have this type of personality, as do 15 percent of people who die of cancer.

Type III individuals are mixed. They bounce between hopelessness and anger. Approximately 9 percent of people who die of cancer or heart disease have a Type III personality.

Type IV individuals are those whom Abraham Maslow would have called self-actualized. These individuals believe happiness is an inside job and approach life with an almost Zenlike sensibility: You cannot make me happy; you cannot make me unhappy. Type IV individuals tend to die of old age or natural causes. *Fewer than*

1 percent of individuals who die of cancer or heart disease have a basic Type IV personality. This is definitely the personality characteristic that you want to cultivate!

IN A GIVEN YEAR IN THE UNITED STATES, AT LEAST 20 percent of individuals are on a prescribed antidepressant drug regimen. But, in fact, it is widely estimated that this number represents less than half of truly depressed people who should be treated. On the surface, it may seem that this "silent majority" is in need of medication; however, the results of treatment with antidepressant drugs are appallingly poor. The best antidepressants have a success rate of approximately 42 percent.

According to the 2005 *Physicians' Desk Reference* (pp. 1585–90), Paxil has a 25 percent success rate at a 20-mg. dose, a 42 percent success rate at a 40-mg. dose, and a 44 percent success rate at a 60-mg. dose (60 mg. is very poorly tolerated!). The "side effects" included nausea in 26 percent of patients, somnolence in 23 percent, dry mouth in 18 percent, constipation in 14 percent, diarrhea in 12 percent, dizziness in 13 percent, insomnia in 13 percent, male genital disorders (including ejaculatory problems) in 23 percent, asthenia in 15 percent, and headache in 18 percent. The results with Prozac® and Effexor® are not much different.

More than thirty years ago, recognizing the significant complications of antidepressant drugs and their low success rate, I began looking for effective and safe alternatives for patients dealing with depression. Having seen some thirty thousand individuals suffering from chronic pain and depression, I have found that by using the most sophisticated test for depression, the **Minnesota Multiphasic Personality Inventory (MMPI)**, 91 percent of these individuals were suffering from significant depression, and that this 91 percent also had significant abnormalities on the scales of hypochondria and hysteria. Indeed, the 9 percent of individuals with chronic pain who did not show depression often appeared to be the most manipulative individuals who often had strong secondary gain—that is, they had reasons not to get well, either because of a pending legal suit such as an automobile accident or a worker's compensation case or they had other psychological abnormalities such as paranoia, schizoid behavior, psychopathic deviancy, or other conditions.

My earliest study of these pain patients with chronic depression consisted just of measuring the twenty-four-hour breakdown component of **serotonin, 5-hydroxyindoleacetic acid (5-HIAA)**, a monamine neurotransmitter that figures largely into the biochemistry of anxiety and depression. I found that 40 percent of these patients were producing an excess of 5-HIAA, and 40 percent actually had a deficient level of DHEA. Using the **Liss stimulator***— an instrument that has come to be known as the Liss cranial electrical stimulator—I found that within two weeks the twenty-four-hour production of serotonin had returned to normal. That is, those who had a low level came up to normal and those at a high level came down to normal. Interestingly, success in dealing with

---

*The **Liss stimulator** is a totally safe device using between 1 and 2 milliamps of current with a repetition rate of 15,000 cycles per second. It has been modified also to have a 500-pulse-per-second and a 15-pulse-per-second modulation of the 15,000 pulses per second. One of the great benefits of this device is that it appears to go through bone. It produces very little sensory stimulation. In fact, at 1 or 2 milliamps, most individuals feel nothing. It does elicit a visual flicker response when it is applied anywhere on the head. We do not know why it works, but it is safe and I have found the Liss, modified to the Shealy specifications, namely a one-hour output, to be more effective than any other known intervention in restoring serotonin and beta-endorphin production.

these chronically ill individuals—who had usually had, at that time, five to seven unsuccessful operations under their belts and been taking multiple medications—turned out to be 80 percent. It was the 20 percent of individuals who had a relatively normal production of serotonin who represented the failure. Incidentally, it does not mean that they did not have pain or that they were not depressed. It is just that the serotonin mechanism was not a major factor here.

The next study involved using just the Liss cranial electrical stimulator in individuals who were chronically depressed, not necessarily with chronic pain but individuals whose depression had not responded to one or more antidepressant medications. In a study of twenty-four such individuals, within two weeks twelve had come out of their depression using nothing but the Liss stimulator transcranially for one hour each morning.

PHOTOSTIMULATION

Shortly after I began using the Liss stimulator in 1975, I also began using pulsed photostimulation. In the 1950s, it was discovered that flashing lights could help put individuals into a hypnotic trance. A number of scientific articles reported that therapists using this approach were able to help individuals lower blood pressure, require less anesthesia for surgery, and use other such helpful procedures with less or without medication. As mentioned in the last chapter, low-frequency photostimulation helps the individual enter a state of relaxation necessary for that needed thirty to forty minutes of deep relaxation a day. I have used photostimulation for thirty years in assisting my patients to relax.

In administering the light therapy, I found that it was most easily accomplished with a specific photostimulator—mine is called the Shealy RelaxMate II™. It allows the client to choose the frequency of photostimulation from anywhere between one and seven cycles per second. A client can also blend blue and red colored lights.

Ninety percent of individuals report feeling deeply relaxed within ten minutes of use of the RelaxMate II™. This adjunct is particularly useful in depressed patients as well as those with anxiety. By this time, I knew that the combined approach of education, cranial electrical stimulation, and photostimulation was helpful in treating patients with chronic pain and/or depression.

Therefore, a two-week program was created: For four hours each day individuals were given one hour of transcranial stimulation with the Liss stimulator, one-hour of photostimulation, a one hour lecture on various aspects of health psychology, and one hour on a vibrating music bed. The latter was added because music is an adjunct in relaxing and to some extent it helps people bring up unfinished emotional trauma so that they can deal with it. This four-hour program, five days a week for two weeks, resulted in 85 percent of the patients coming out of their depression.

QUARTZ CRYSTALS

Quartz crystal has a piezoelectric effect, which means that it stores electromagnetic energy. It both receives and transmits electromagnetic energy. Interestingly, our body is a giant electromagnetic energetic device. The skeleton, muscles, tendons, and intestines are all piezoelectric. Thus, it appears that crystals, properly mentally programmed, can have a beneficial effect upon health.

In 1988, I was asked to investigate the use of quartz crystals. I integrated this investigation into my four-part study outlined above, comparing the efficacy of storage of electromagnetic energy in quartz versus glass crystals. On the last day of the two weeks, in a double-blind study so that both the nurse distributing the crystals and the patients did not know whether they were getting a glass or a quartz crystal, each individual was given either a quartz or a glass crystal. Each crystal was passed through a candle to "release" any stored electromagnetic energy. The individuals then held it in the palms of their hands while blowing into it and willing their own personal healing phrase, such as "I am happy, active, and comfortable." They then wore the crystal in a pouch around their neck for the next three months. Each morning at home they were to "reprogram" the crystal daily for one week and then once a week thereafter. They were also given a twenty-minute tape of the music that they had used during the program to use at home. (I had chosen for that particular music experience either classical music—Beethoven's Sixth Symphony, Pachelbel's Canon in D, or Mozart's *Requiem*—or *Best of Kitaro*, Bearns and Dexter's *Golden Voyage*, vol. 4, *Spectrum Suite* by Steven Halpern, or Aeoliah's *The Seven Chakras: Crystal Illumination*.)

Other than the education, music, and the crystal to use at home, no further therapy was used. When the individuals returned three months later, only 28 percent of the patients who had received the glass had remained out of depression, but a striking 70 percent of those who had received the quartz crystal had remained undepressed.

By this time I knew that the Liss cranial stimulator could relieve depression in 50 percent of individuals with no other intervention (10 percent better than the best antidepressant drugs—and without any complications), and I knew that the Liss stimulator, the use of photostimulation, plus education and vibratory music could assist in relaxation. And now I knew that quartz crystal could help 70 percent maintain free of depression, with no further intervention. It is important to remember that all the patients with depression with whom I have worked had already failed to respond to one or several antidepressant drugs.

In the long run, it is infinitely less expensive and more effective for individuals to use a Liss stimulator than it is to use any antidepressant drug. If patients are willing to combine use of the stimulator with photostimulation for relaxation, listening to good music, and getting some education, it appears that most people would respond well to this treatment approach without any complications.*

DEPRESSION AND AMINO ACIDS

In one of my studies of depressed individuals, I found that an incredible *100 percent* of them are deficient in one to seven of the essential amino acids. The essential amino acids are: **histidine, isoleucine, leucine, lysine, methionine, phenylalanine, threonine, tryptophan, taurine,** and **valine.** Eighty-six percent of the individuals were deficient in taurine, usually the most abundant amino acid in the human body. Taurine is synergistic with magnesium. Both magnesium and taurine keep the electrical charge stable on the cell.

---

*Incidentally, anxiety—even very severe cases of anxiety—also responds well to this approach. In one other study where I used electrical stimulation with the SheLi TENS™ on the Ring of Fire (see chapter 2), the twelve specific acupuncture points for raising DHEA, I also got a 70 percent improvement in depression.

Replacing taurine can be helpful but, in general, individuals deficient in taurine tend to be deficient in more than one amino acid. It is fairly easy to get the taurine you need by preparing a meat broth. In fact, this simple broth will provide you with more amino acids than just taurine alone.

MEAT BROTH FOR TAURINE DEFICIENCIES

- To prepare meat broth, place 8 ounces of any kind of meat cut into small squares into a Crock-Pot or slow cooker with 1 quart of water, seasoned with soy sauce and onion, carrot, celery, or other vegetables to give it good flavor, and 2 tablespoons of vinegar. Cook on low heat for 8 to 12 hours.
- Drink a pint of this broth each day for a month, then one cup a day long-term. It may well be that depressed individuals have difficulty breaking down protein adequately, so the meat broth helps break down the protein and release amino acids that are easily assimilated. Actually, drinking meat broth is a lot cheaper than taking a lot of the amino-acid supplements, and it also tastes good!

FAMILY, LOVE, AND OTHER
ADJUNCTS FOR MENTAL HEALTH

It pays to have a nurturing atmosphere.[72] Marriage contributes years of life only to men, which indicates a strong relationship between emotional support systems and psychological well-being. The strength of relationships between children and parents has been shown to be predictive of cancer. Those who did not have a close relationship with their parents—those without a sense of nurturance—had a much higher incidence of cancer than those who had closeness with parents.[73]

Negative attitude and lack of a supportive personal relationship are among the most damaging factors to health in general. Studies have found that **immune dysregulation** occurs, and a wide variety of "conditions associated with aging" are increased, including heart disease, osteoporosis, arthritis, Type 2 diabetes, and many cancers. Chronic low-grade infections are also more common.[74] Negative emotions have further been associated with Alzheimer's disease, periodontal disease, and generalized frailty.[75]

MENOPAUSE AND ANDROPAUSE:
CONTRIBUTORS TO DEPRESSION

Most people are familiar with the major hormonal shift that occurs in women usually around the age of fifty. But in fact, a similar change takes place in both men and women in the hypothalamic pituitary control center for regulation of all hormones. In women, the **gonadal dysfunction** is largely cessation of ovulation and a marked decrease in production of **estrogen** and **progesterone**.

Menopause is generally understood to occur in all women. **Andropause,** on the other hand, is a similar hormonal decline in men, occurring at roughly the same age as menopause in women. In men, the major gonadal decrease is in production of **testosterone,** especially "free" testosterone. In addition, the normal circadian rhythm of testosterone production is lost. Another major factor contributing to the decline in male health is an increase in **IL-6/ interleukin-6** (discussed in detail later.)

Again, this is a problem found in both men and women as IL-6, an inflammation-provoking **cytokinase,** is ordinarily suppressed by estrogen and testosterone. High levels of IL-6 lead to increased chronic inflammatory disease, decrease in body mass, loss of bone, low-grade anemia, decreased serum albumin and cholesterol, and increased inflammatory protein such as C-reactive protein (CRP), which has been highly associated with coronary artery disease, as well as serum amyloid A, which has been widely correlated with Alzheimer's disease. The age-associated increase in IL-6 has also been linked to lymphoplastic diseases such as multiple myeloma. There is also a strong association between decreasing DHEA and lowered testosterone. In fact, the decline in DHEA is significantly greater than that of testosterone.

All these, but most particularly low testosterone levels, are associated with sarcopenia and loss of muscle mass, resulting in increases in fat even in nonobese individuals. The thinning of hair, depression, impaired sleep patterns, and impaired changes in insulin resistance are all part of the adverse effects of decreased levels of testosterone.

Just as women begin in their thirties missing some ovulations during their menstrual cycles, the actual beginning decrease in testosterone level takes place by age forty in most men. These problems are extremely universal in human beings, with similar findings reported from Korea, Nigeria, Poland, Germany, China, Great Britain, and other countries.

One of the greatest controversies associated with the changes in levels of testosterone in men is the relationship to **prostate disease.** One of greatest contributors to prostate disease is obesity. There is, unequivocally, an inverse relationship between the production of testosterone and excess body weight. Anyone with a Body Mass Index (BMI) of 25 or above should lose weight to somewhere between the 19 and 24 BMI level, both for prostate health as well as for health in general. Both benign prostatic hypertrophy and prostate cancer are believed by some specialists to be aggravated if men are given testosterone supplements. However, a few researchers argue that giving testosterone actually might inhibit prostate enlargement and/or cancer. One of the most fascinating associations with increased prostate disease is the association of a low level of vitamin D with increased prostate cancer. Low vitamin D is also associated with many immune problems, including skin and colon cancers.

From the point of view of the male psyche, perhaps the most critical psychosocial change at this time is decreasing erectile function, which varies tremendously and is much more prevalent than is generally believed. Again, it begins as early as the mid-thirties in some men and, relative to virtual total impotence or erectile dysfunction, as it is currently called, occurs in the majority of men by age eighty. The widespread use of Viagra®, even among young men, attests to this particular concern and, although some younger men use it primarily to last longer or to shorten the refractory period, it is not uncommon for men in their forties to find it useful for the beginning problems of erectile dysfunction.

Since both the quality of life and indeed the length of life are strongly correlated with decreasing levels of testosterone and the resultant physical disability including great frailty that occurs in aging men, some attention to this disorder needs to be given by virtually all men—and their spouses! Based upon the virtual certainty in difficulty as you mature, here are my recommendations:

RECOMMENDATIONS FOR MEN IN MIDDLE AGE

Beginning at age forty:

• Get a salivary hormone test for: *cortisol, testosterone, DHEA or DHEA sulfate,* and *estrone.*

If all your levels are in the middle to upper part of the so-called normal range, just keep up good health habits. If you have no symptoms, repeat this battery of tests at age fifty.

No later than age fifty:

• If there are no urinary-tract symptoms, begin taking beta sitosterol, 1,200 mg. per day.
• After age fifty, men should be getting 1,000 units of vitamin D and 3 mg. of boron daily.

The important information about the prostate, from my point of view is "If it ain't broke, don't try to fix it." The evidence is quite strong that unless one has symptoms, it is better not to go mucking around with invasive procedures, especially needle biopsies. The most likely way to prevent problems is to follow the program outlined above. Surgery is something that should be considered only when there are significant symptoms, as I am not at all impressed that "early" surgery is worthwhile; it inevitably leads to total impotence that is not treatable by anything except surgery with an implantable device!

Obviously if DHEA levels are in the lower half of the normal range or below, it is already time to start on DHEA restoration, as outlined in chapter 2.

For those of you with erectile dysfunction, consider taking the following:

- *Tribulus terrestris* (a Chinese herb), 500 mg. up to eight daily
- Timed Release Arginine, 1,000 mg. twice a day
- *Epimedium sagittatum* (an herbal supplement, also called horny goat weed), 100 mg. up to six daily

One of the first things to use in treating erectile dysfunction is **natural progesterone cream,** one-quarter teaspoon twice a day on the skin. This both helps restore DHEA and appears to increase libido in many men. It also blocks **5-alpha reductase,** the enzyme that converts testosterone to dihydrotestosterone. It is dihydrotestosterone that is thought to be at least partially responsible for benign prostatic hypertrophy and prostate cancer.

Beyond this, before going to one of the pharmaceutical products, try **VigEros**™, which contains both **cnidium monnier** and **xanthoparmelia scabrosa**. If four days of these treatments do not help and you have had an adequate physical exam to rule out serious problems such as diabetes with peripheral neuropathy or atherosclerosis, and assuming that you are not on any cardiac or any hypertensive drugs, consider one of the erectile dysfunction drugs. The three now on the market are Cialis®, Levitra®, and Viagra®. Cialis® appears to be best. I am currently evaluating an electromagnetic device that, with the herbal formula mentioned earlier, may be as good as the drugs and much safer.

MENOPAUSE

By their mid-thirties, women begin to miss an occasional ovulation. By the time onset of menopause occurs, estrogen production is markedly diminished, as is progesterone production. These endocrine changes may cause severe hot flashes, marked mood changes, irritation and depression, insomnia, loss of libido, memory loss, etc. It is at this time of life that many women opt for hormone-replacement therapy. But this type of drug-dependent therapy comes at a risk.

Women with low levels of IGF-1/Insulinlike Growth Factor-1 (which promotes growth) and high levels of IL-6/Interleukin-6 (a chemical related to the family of interleukins, which cause inflammation) are at a greater risk of disability, and even death. Having both a low IGF-1 and a high IL-6 causes aggregate dysregulation or maladaptation in both the general endocrine and immune systems.[76] IGF-1 deficiency is also involved in cognitive deficits associated with aging, for example in Alzheimer's disease.

The level of IGF-1 directly relates to one's memory, intelligence, and ability to process information; and those with the lowest level of IGF-1 have a high level of mental disability. IGF-1 levels below 9.4 nmol/L are negatively associated with level and decline of information-processing speed.[77] Body fat is also significantly associated with IGF-1 levels. This is particularly true of trunk fat, which is a significant correlate of low IGF-1 levels.

Although this hasn't reached the national news media as well as other studies related to it have, women taking horse estrogen, Premarin® and Provera®, have much lower levels of IGF-1. This is at least one biochemical measurement that gives us some evidence of one of the reasons that **HRT (hormone replacement therapy)** has shortened life expectancy in women.[78]

SUGGESTIONS
FOR MENOPAUSAL WOMEN

- If you have not suffered cancer of the breast, ovaries, or uterus, natural progesterone is by far the best supplement, in one-quarter-tsp doses applied on the skin, twice daily.
- If you are experiencing symptoms such as nervousness, irritability, severe hot flashes, and insomnia, take *black cohosh* and *dong quai*, available in many different herbal combinations.
- If black cohosh and dong quai do not alleviate symptoms, consider visiting a compounding pharmacy for a combination of 2.5 mg. of Biest (equal amounts of estriol and

estradiol) and 60 mg. of natural progesterone in a daily dose of 2 applications of one-quarter teaspoon, as outlined above.

- I strongly recommend against taking under any circumstance Estrone, Premarin®, or any of the artificial progesterones, especially Provera® and Prempro®.*
- 1,000 mg. of vitamin D
- 1.5 grams of calcium as citrate or Calcium Plus 500
- Biogenics® Magnesium Lotion, at least 2 to 4 teaspoons a day, depending on weight
- 3 mg. of boron a day
- Women with a tendency toward *fibrocystic breast disease* or fibroids also need to consider an adequate supplement of *iodine,* which is probably a minimum of 750 mcg. and up to 12.5 mg daily.
- A BMI between 19 and 24 (See Figure 4.1, Body Mass Index Chart.)
- Adequate exercise
- Positive mental attitude!

*Statistically, these drugs produce a significant increase in cancer and stroke and provide no help for osteoporosis. Unless you weigh eight hundred pounds, you should never consider Premarin® in the first place. It is horse, not human, estrogen!

BODY MASS INDEX CHART													
	5'0"	5'1"	5'2"	5'3"	5'4"	5'5"	5'6"	5'7"	5'8"	5'9"	5'10"	5'11"	6'0"
100	19	18	18	17	17								
110	21	20	20	19	19	18	18	17					
120	23	22	22	21	20	20	19	19	18	17	17		
130	25	24	24	23	22	22	21	20	20	19	18		
140	27	26	26	25	24	23	23	22	21	21	20	19	19
150	29	28	28	27	26	25	24	23	23	22	21	20	20
160	31	30	29	28	27	27	26	25	24	24	23	22	22
170	33	32	31	30	29	28	28	26	26	25	24	23	23
180	35	34	33	32	31	30	29	28	28	27	26	25	25
190	37	36	35	34	33	31	31	29	29	28	27	27	26
200	39	38	37	36	34	33	32	31	30	30	29	28	27
210	41	40	39	37	36	35	34	33	32	31	30	30	29
220	42	42	41	39	38	37	36	34	33	33	32	31	30
230	45	44	43	41	40	39	37	36	35	34	33	32	31
240	47	46	45	43	41	40	39	38	37	36	35	34	33

Figure 4.1

Ultimately, everything is related to everything. Depression is a common disease, for which alternative, complementary, and holistic therapies are highly superior to pharmaceuticals. Similarly, menopause and andropause, normal physiological changes, are usually well managed with safer **complementary-alternative-medicine (CAM)** approaches. *See Chapter 7.*

5

ELECTRICAL CONCEPTS OF ENERGY AND ELECTROMAGNETISM

Conventional medicine has ignored bioelectricity for almost a century, choosing to focus on chemistry. The truth is that we can no longer afford to cultivate the concept of a separation between biochemistry, physical anatomy, and **electromagnetism.** We are electrochemical beings, and electricity invariably produces electromagnetism.

Electromagnetic frequency is energy that moves through space by electric or magnetic waves. The electromagnetic spectrum involves electrical waves that move in planes perpendicular to magnetic ones. The electrical wave produces magnetic ones, and moving magnetic waves produce electrical ones. Some of the common known waves are listed in the following chart.

FREQUENCY IN CYCLES PER SECOND

X-rays	10^{18} (1 billion billion)
Ultraviolet/visible light	10^{16} (10 million billion)
Radar	10^{10} (10 billion)
UHF, UVF, FM, AM radio	10^{6} (1 million)
Human DNA	54 to 78 times 10^{9}
	(54 to 78 billion)

A portrait of what we have referred to as spirit not only exists but is most tangibly expressed in or through the electromagnetic bioenergetic framework. Our evolving knowledge allows us to break down the usual perception of reality that the tangible physical comes first and is dominant over energy. Energy is indeed the basic framework, and its study is the science of life and consciousness. This means the time has come to base our concept of health on the human body and spirit as co-creators. A model of health consciousness needs to reflect the fact that the human spirit is connected with the body through the electromagnetic field. Indeed, as I will emphasize many times, electromagnetic energy can elicit, control, and trigger biological changes, both chemically and mentally.

THE ELECTROMAGNETIC
FRAMEWORK OF LIFE

The concept of electricity and magnetism was first discussed in 1600 in William Gilbert's *De Magnete*. He established the difference between electricity (he coined the word) and magnetism, and he introduced the concept of magnetic fields. Even throughout the seventeenth century, however, scientists such as Descartes and William Harvey believed that an "animating force" or "vital spirit" was necessary for the mechanical physics of the body. Otto von Guericke invented the first electric generating device in 1660. Newton theorized that Descartes' vital principle, or animating force, was an "all pervading ether," which not only filled the universe but also flowed through nerves to produce the functions we call life.

Early in the eighteenth century, Stephen Gray discovered that some materials were conductors of electricity. Today we think of copper as an excellent conductor, whereas wood and glass shield or prevent conduction. Shortly thereafter Stephan Hales theorized that nerves might function by conducting electrical impulses.

By the mid-1700s electricity was being artificially generated, stored, and transmitted. This new discovery was quickly applied to treatment of a variety of illnesses, with the first book about it, *Electrical Medicine,* published in 1752 by Johann Schaeffer.

The "proof" of transmission of electricity was not established until 1786, when Luigi Galvani and his associates discovered that external static electricity could travel through a nerve and make a muscle contract. Galvani then decided that "animal electricity" was the long-theorized "vital force."

A nephew of Galvani, Giovanni Aldini, reported significant improvement, then complete rehabilitation, of a schizophrenic with transcranial electrical stimulation!

In 1820, Hans Christian Oersted discovered electromagnetism in demonstrating the effect of electricity upon a compass. Ten years later, Carlo Matteucci first demonstrated that injured tissues generated an electrical current. Pursuing Matteucci's work, DuBois Reymond demonstrated the nerve impulse, the essential mechanism for transfer of information within the nervous system. His colleagues even measured the velocity of a nerve impulse at 30 meters per second. Julius Bernstein in 1868 introduced the concept of bioelectricity, created by transfer of ions across cell membranes. Today we know that intracellular potassium and magnesium are higher than extracellular levels, while extracellular sodium and calcium are higher than intracellular levels. It is the movement of these four ions that creates bioelectricity. With Bernstein's discovery, the machinists of science quickly rejected electricity in favor of the chemical/physics concept, ignoring the fact that the chemical reaction generated electricity!

But clinicians were more pragmatic, and thousands of nineteenth-century physicians used electricity for treatment of a variety of problems, even though science and ultimately medicine rejected electrotherapy in favor of physics and chemistry, after the 1910 publication of the Flexner Report. Abraham Flexner was hired by the American Medical Association to assess medicine in the United States. Although there were undoubtedly nonscientific abuses in the system, Flexner was a machinist supreme and recommended excommunication of every naturalist concept of health. Thus, osteopathy, acupuncture, and homeopathy were targeted, along with some undoubtedly ineffective methods of treatment.

Unfortunately Flexner's report was accepted as law, thereby throwing out the baby with the bathwater. Fifty percent of all medical schools and hospitals were closed. Homeopathy and acupuncture have barely survived. Osteopathy narrowly escaped extinction, and was under constant attack until the mid-1960s when, perhaps, the battle against chiropractic was so strong that the American Medical Association grudgingly accepted osteopathy.

While most aspects of life were improving through advances in electric technology and electrification of the world—lighting, cooking appliances, radio, electric engines, and so on—after 1910 the medical establishment largely ignored both electrotherapy and the potential negative effects of a world with increasing artificially generated electromagnetism.

This medical scientific black hole even ignored such significant findings in Edison's lab as the induction of a subjective sensation of flickering light when human volunteers were placed in an alternating on/off magnetic field. This total denial of any effects of electromagnetic fields on life is particularly hard to reconcile with common sense and logic.

Since chemistry was the lifeline of the cell, biochemistry and chemical drugs became the foundation of modern medicine. In fact, numerous other important electromagnetic experiments were ignored. In 1902, Alphonse Leduc reported narcotizing animals by passing 35 volts of alternating current at 110 cycles per second (1 hertz [Hz]=1 cycle/sec). Ugo Cerletti in 1938 introduced electroshock therapy for schizophrenia and later for depression.

In 1929, Hans Berger discovered the electroencephalogram, which measured the electrical rhythm of the brain; he postulated a "bioelectric field." In the same year the electrocardiogram (EKG or ECG) was discovered; it has been invaluable in the diagnosis of cardiac disease. Later, electromyograms (EMGs) and nerve-conduction testing became essential diagnostic tests for neurology.

In the 1940s, Thomas Hodgkin, Aldous Huxley, and Sir John Eccles demonstrated, through intracellular nerve cell recordings, the generation of electrical discharges by the sodium/potassium exchange. Unfortunately, once again, the mechanists jumped upon the chemical/physical bandwagon and ignored the undeniable essential duality of nerve-cell function—electrical *and* chemical.

Despite the snub by medical science of the underlying bioelectrical life energy, Albert Szent-Györgyi, the Nobel laureate who discovered the biologic oxidation mechanism of vitamin C, mentioned that "some basic fact about life is still missing." His concept that solid-state electronic processes were generated by biologic molecules reawakened a relatively limited but important interest in electrobiology. A number of investigators demonstrated the major influence of DC current (the flow of electric charge) in influencing neuronal behavior and a variety of influences of electricity upon brain function, mood, personality, and sleep. In 1976, D. K. Nias demonstrated in double-blind studies the benefits of electrosleep, already used in the USSR for over twenty-five years at that time.[79] Interestingly, electrosleep did not induce sleep during the application of a very weak electrical current across the head. The treatment was applied in the morning to assist sleep in the evening. This is exactly the same effect I have found with the Liss stimulator, as reported in chapter 4 ("Depression").

Eventually the solid-state electronic activity of the neuron system was proven by Tsuji Ishiko and W. R. Lowenstein's demonstration of electric potential changes induced by raising temperatures without action potential effects in nerve fibers.[80] These and similar DC changes in the eye cannot be explained on the basis of ion exchanges. And indeed, B. B. Libet and R. W. Gerard had reported in the 1940s electrical brain current of a nonionic nature, that which today would be called "displacement current." As stated earlier, most brain activity is created by intracellular to extracellular (and vice versa) movement of sodium, potassium, calcium, and magnesium ions.

In the 1960s, Robert Becker and co-workers demonstrated that currents of only 30 microamps could induce loss of consciousness and general anesthesia in salamanders. And they found that field strengths of 3,000 gauss, oriented 90 degrees in a fronto-occipital vector, produced similar results.[81] Later experiments demonstrated a magnetic field around the head, with eventual development of a magnetoencephalogram.

Concomitantly Becker resurrected experiments of the first decade of the twentieth century, using electrical current to assist in regeneration of tissue regrowth of limbs or tails in salamanders and even of the forearm, but not paws, of cats. His work later led to the development of electrical current for improved healing of fractures of various bones. Becker believes that "intrinsic electromagnetic energy inherent in the nervous system of the body is therefore the factor that exerts the major controlling influence over growth processes in general."[82] Indeed, Becker believes this electromagnetic property is "intrinsic" in all living tissues.

The piezoelectronic property of bone was established in 1954. The piezoelectric mechanism is that production of an electrical stimulus evoked by mechanical stress or pressure. Indeed, piezoelectric properties even of collagen, the universal "glue" substance of the body, were established by Becker. And bone, dentin, tendon, aorta, trachea, intestines, elastin, and nucleic acids are all "normal" human anatomical "transducers" of piezoelectro-energy. Carrying this correlation of living tissue to electrical phenomena even further, super conductivity, once thought to be associated only with metals at very low temperature, has been demonstrated in frog sciatic nerve, growth of bacteria, production of carbon dioxide by yeast, division in sea urchin eggs, and in cholates (normal bile salts).

Becker's work within living systems led him eventually to study the linkage between "artificial" external electromagnetic fields and the "normal" bioelectromagnetics of life itself. Electromagnetic energy influences the piezoelectric property of tissue to emit phonons, sound waves with a wave length low enough to resonate with cell membranes.[83]

Indeed it is this bioelectromagnetic aspect that is largely responsible for known and unknown biological cycles or clocks, most well known as the circadian or diurnal rhythm (variations during night and day, the twenty-four-hour variations). These rhythms are very subtle.

In 1954, Frank Brown of Northwestern University demonstrated that oysters moved from New Hampshire to Evanston, Illinois, changed their opening and closing to coincide with tides even while at Evanston, as if it were a seacoast.[84] Similarly, human beings transported great distances longitudinally change the night-day timing of many neurochemicals, such as blood levels of cortisol. In general, this change is accomplished at a rate of about one hour per day. Thus, a trip from New York to Australia requires at least seven days for biologic accommodation. One of the most critical changes is that of production of melatonin, essential for good sleep. Thus, "jet lag" may be the most widely recognized negative effect of electromagnetic distortion in today's fast-paced world. In a sense, such "artificial" rapid change in natural electromagnetic fields is a twentieth-century development.

. . .

WE GENERALLY CONSIDER LIFE TO INCLUDE HUMANS, animals, plants, amoebae, and even bacteria, fungi, and viruses. But what allows bacteria or humans to "live"? In one of the oldest continuing civilizations, China, life is considered to be the result of chi or qi. One Western scientist, Wilhelm Reich, one of the few noted psychiatrists either to consider life energy or to study it scientifically, called life energy "orgone." A Russian engineer, Georges Lakhovsky, who published *The Secret of Life* over seventy years ago, stated that human DNA resonates at 50+ billion cycles per second.[85]

Modern Ukrainian quantum physicists have taken Lakhovsky's concepts much further. They state that human DNA vibrates at 54 to 78 gigahertz (billions of cycles per second); animals at 47 gigahertz; and plants at 42 gigahertz. They believe that each individual resonates most significantly at a unique "eigen" frequency. Thus, there could be 27 billion specific frequencies (i.e., those between 54 and 78 gigahertz). Interestingly, these physicists believe that each organ collectively projects its vector, or energy, along a specific pathway for that organ, the **acupuncture meridian** for that organ. Thus, modern physics is providing a foundation for integrating ancient wisdom, acupuncture, and quantum theory.

In December 1992, I spent twelve days embarking upon my initial study of **giga-energy** in Kiev. That study led to my intuitive reception of the Ring of Fire (discussed in chapter 2). During my visit to Kiev, I was trained in the technology of the Ukraine physicists who had taken Lakhovsky's concepts to new heights. When I returned to the United States, I quickly learned that Americans did not want to be microwaved! So I coined the term **GigaTENS** for these frequencies.

Over a five-year period, as I explored this technology, I intuitively perceived five significant circuits in the human body. Over the next five years I discovered that four of these circuits specifically raised DHEA, **Aldosterone, Neurotensin,** or Calcitonin. The fifth lowered free radicals. Because of their clear modulation of life energy, I consider these pathways to be the **Sacred Rings of Life.** I named them Fire, Water, Air, Earth, and Crystal. As outlined in an earlier chapter, recharging these circuits is done with another of my inventions, the SheLi TENS™, which is the only American device that includes DNA frequencies of 54 to 78 GigaHz.

Over the past thirty years, extensive work has demonstrated natural electromagnetic phenomena involved in the migration of birds, fish, and even honeybees. Even some bacteria orient themselves to the earth's magnetic field, apparently because they contain microcrystals of magnetite (the smallest known unit of magnetism). Only within the past two years have similar crystals been found in the human brain. Interestingly, humans appear to have some electromagnetic "tracking" sense that is disrupted when magnets of 140 to 300 gauss are applied to their heads. American eels are affected by DC electrical fields of 0.67 microvolts/cm. and currents of 0.00167 microamps/cm.^{2}, truly subtle influences.

At the other extreme of "artificial" electromagnetic effects, we now know that electric blankets are extremely dangerous to the fetus in pregnant women, with marked increases in miscarriage and malformations.

Central to understanding **bioelectromagnetism** is the 7-to-10-Hz frequency, which is the dominant rhythm of the earth and the common frequency of the EEG of all higher animals and humans. When people are removed from the normal 7-to-10-Hz background and placed in specially shielded rooms, their EEGs, mood, and diurnal neurochemistry change. Similarly, cumulative external electromagnetic influences can affect mood, sleep, health, and even one's EEG. The EEGs of patients who are significantly depressed show significant asymmetry, most often excess activity in the right frontal lobe; inability to follow flickering light frequency; inappropriate EEG (excess speeding up or slowing down with flickering lights); and abnormal EEG activity even with an electric clock near the head. These individuals sometimes become so sensitive that radio waves may disturb their ability to function mentally or intellectually. Meanwhile, humans in underground electromagnetically shielded rooms become destabilized and desynchronized; 10-Hz electrical fields assist them in returning to normal diurnal patterns.[86]

EEG changes, as well as diurnal rhythms, have been induced by magnetism of only 1 to 3 minutes at 200 to 1,000 gauss, as well as to **electromagnetic frequencies (EMF)** of 3 to 50 Hz. Pulsed EMFs have also been reported to affect evoked potential of neuronal firing behavior as well as response to drugs. Such effects may occur at levels of EMFs as low as 30 microwatts/cm^2. Even in tissue culture, brain-tissue production of norepinephrine can be affected by minute amounts of electromagnetic energy.

Animals exposed to higher levels of energy such as 200 to 300 gauss for seventy hours show major anatomical damage of brain tissue. Even 60 microwatts/cm^2 of 3 GHz energy applied for up to six weeks can cause brain damage. Biological effects can occur at electromagnetic levels well below thermal energy.

Aggression, avoidance, and sleep patterns of animals are susceptible to EMFs. In humans, reaction time is affected by pulsed magnetic fields. Even 1 gauss of 60 Hz can alter the ability of humans to concentrate. Extremely low EMFs of 0.00001 volts can alter EEGs.[87]

In other words, *applied electromagnetic energy can elicit, control, or trigger biological changes.* Becker has emphasized that electromagnetic fields can be stressors. Adrenal production of cortisol is significantly altered by pulsed electromagnetic energy: The effect is dependent upon field strength, frequency, duration of exposure, continuous versus intermittent exposure, and even biochemical individuality.[88] The thyroid, pancreas, and adrenal glands are all affected by EMFs.

In nonendocrine tissues, the rhythm of the heart can be easily altered by EMFs. At extremely low levels, EMFs of 25 to 50 microwatts/cm^2 can change white blood cells dramatically. Robert Becker and G. Selden conclude that "there is no biological function which can be said to be impervious to non-thermal EMFs— they are a fundamental and pervasive factor in the biology of every living organism."[89]

Today because of television, radio, microwaves, radar, and satellites, human-made "artificial" EMFs overwhelmingly dominate the normal background of "Earth's" electromagnetic environment. Today almost all areas of the world have electric fields of 0.10/m. or greater, or magnetic ones of 100 microgauss or more. Average exposures may be 8 to 10 times these fields. In the former Soviet Union, "safe" exposure is felt to be below 1 microwatt/cm^2. The ultimate epidemiologic health effects of such massive change in environmental EMFs will not be easily known for many years.

Meanwhile, beneficial therapeutic effects of applied EMFs are increasing. Perhaps the most pervasive use has been cardiac pacing, where millions of lives have been gratifyingly and effectively prolonged by pacemakers. Pain control through TENS (transcutaneous electrical nerve stimulator units—electroacupuncture) is also at the forefront of bioelectromagnetic therapy. Treatment of depression and restoration of neurochemical homeostasis is the work to which we turn our attention in this book. The devices used are currently well within the safety guidelines of the U.S. government, and the benefits seem so great, in many instances, that it appears wise to consider them.

ELECTROPHYSIOLOGY AND SEX

Earlier work on electrophysiology is also of interest. Wilhelm Reich set out to answer the question of whether sexual orgasm was "an essentially mechanical process."[90] In the early days of mechanistic dominance, many people apparently considered orgasm to be simply a "mechanical" release. This limited mechanistic view even led psychiatrists to conclude it was not natural for women to experience orgasm since they had no "mechanical release" or ejaculation! Reich felt that orgiastic potency was the key to understanding emotional life in general and psychic disorders, neuroses, in particular. Thus, Reich assumed that sexual tension and relaxation require a "bioelectrical discharge" during orgasm. Reich noted that genital friction led to involuntary genital muscle contracture, greater with gentle, slow friction than vigorous, rapid friction. He believed that strongly muscularly armored (blocked) individuals preferred vigorous movement and were vegetatively inhibited.

Reich claimed that the "basic function of all living matter, namely tension and relaxation, charge and discharge," were part of the natural function of orgasm. Thus orgiastic bioelectric discharge produced pleasure and relaxation; blocking such discharge caused tension, anxiety, and separation from the partner. Thus, he considered orgasm "one of the most important modal points of the body-soul problem."[91]

In orgiastic function the first requirement is vegetative excitation and increased blood filling of genitals, a parasympathetic effect, producing increased genital tone. Sympathetic anxious excitation leads to constricture of arteries and decreased blood flow. Thus, increased tension during sexual excitation has a direct mechanical basis. But voluntary tensing of the genital muscles impedes gratification.

Reich noted that the involuntary muscle tension created by genital friction was the same as that created by electrically stimulating muscles. Eventually the friction leads to muscle clonus, involuntary automatic contractions concomitant with orgasm. The mechanical friction/tension builds an electrical charge that must lead to both mechanical and electrical discharge. He insisted that postorgasmic relaxation was not mechanical but bioelectric.

Thus, he considered the normal natural process of orgasm to be tension—discharge—relaxation, the centerpiece of his concept of expansion/contraction as the governing principle in life itself. "Mechanical tension leads to an electrical discharge, and electrical discharge leads to mechanical relaxation."[92] He felt this link between mechanics and electricity was also the distinguishing characteristic of living matter—but of course piezoelectricity is not necessarily living!

Reich emphasized that the sympathetic system acts like calcium, producing tension, whereas the parasympathetic system acts like potassium, leading to relaxation. He further believed that cholesterol is like calcium and lecithin like potassium. Alkalines behave like potassium and acids like calcium. These correlations are important, as it is the sympathetic/parasympathetic balance that determines total ability to handle stress. And the balance of calcium, potassium, and magnesium is a critical factor in stress reactions.

There is an antithesis between sexuality and anxiety: the parasympathetic leads to peripheral excitation and central relaxation of sexual expansion; the sympathetic leads to peripheral relaxation and central excitation or anxiety. Electrical discharge in muscles leads to mechanical relaxation. As mechanical muscle tension builds, the piezoelectric effect increases the voltage gradient. At some critical gradient, electrical overload occurs, leading to that electrical discharge.

Sexual excitation is an electrical charging of the erogenous surface (genitals, etc.), and orgasm is a discharge of the potential accumulated during stimulation/activation. "Orgasm is a basic manifestation of living substance and the tension-charge formula cannot be applied to nonliving nature."[93]

Skin response to emotions is best measured through changes in electrical potential and resistance. "The electrical function of sexual zones is different from that of the rest of the skin."[94] Sexual skin (genitals, tongue, lips, nipples, ears) has either much higher or lower potential than nonsexual skin. "Muscular motor activity in general and rhythmic friction, the rubbing together of pleasurably excitable body surfaces, are the fundamental biological phenomena of sexuality."[95] Friction without pleasure does not increase potential; friction with pleasure does. In anxiety or annoyance, surface potential decreases.

Reich believed that the vegetative muscle system is the generation of bioelectrical energy in the human body. Since sexually responsive skin is the only skin that responds with marked increase in potential, he concluded that sexual activity is the bioenergetic productive process itself.

From Reich to Becker, and from many other current investigators, we know now that electromagnetism is the currently measurable energetic foundation for life energy itself. Although metaphysically oriented individuals describe a fifth-dimensional energetic system, there is currently no *measured* fifth-dimensional alternative energy system. Ultimately, mentally, the *function* of the body is electromagnetic and electromagnetically controllable. Someday we will harness this fifth-dimensional energy, often called love, and have ultimate control. Meanwhile we must deal with electrobiology, diagnostically and therapeutically.

6

CHEMICAL AND ELECTROMAGNETIC ASPECTS OF HEALTH AND DISEASE

The increase in "artificial electromagnetic energy" (especially our sixty-cycle electrical grid and machines) present in the modern world has produced some significant illnesses, not the least of which is **chronic fatigue.** Chronic fatigue syndrome has presented one of the more controversial illnesses of the last decade, but it appears to have existed even in the last century, although it was less common then. One hundred years ago it was called neurasthenia. Indeed, none other than Florence Nightingale probably suffered from this syndrome. Other diagnoses, including Wilson's disease, chronic Epstein-Barr, candidiasis, environmental sensitivity, and myeloencephalopathy have also been used to describe this confusing and much-maligned array of symptoms. I propose integrating this dazzling array into one comprehensive diagnosis, *Electromagnetic Dysthymia* (EMD).

DIAGNOSTIC FEATURES OF ELECTROMAGNETIC DYSTHYMIA

- Chronic fatigue
- Various immune symptoms (multiple allergies, myelo-encephalopathy, chronic Epstein-Barr, candidiasis)
- Depression
- 30 or more symptoms*
- DHEA less than 450 in a man; less than 350 in a woman
- Deficient intracellular magnesium
- Deficiency in one or more essential amino acids
- EEG brain map abnormalities
- Asymmetry
- Failure to follow flashing lights (photostimulation)†
- Inappropriate response to photofrequency
- Abnormal hypersensitivity to minor electromagnetic exposure, such as an electrical clock within 6 inches of the head

*A symptom is a feeling, sensation, or awareness that something is "wrong" with the physical body.

† In nondepressed individuals, the electrical rhythm of the brain adjusts to increase the frequency that is flashed by a light into the eyes.

ESSENTIAL CLINICAL FEATURES OF ELECTROMAGNETIC DYSTHYMIA

CHRONIC FATIGUE SYNDROME

- fatigue
- lack of energy
- poor-quality sleep (but need for more sleep/rest than normal)
- anxiety
- irritability
- weakness

These symptoms alone may be found in many chronic illnesses and, of course, comprehensive diagnostic testing must be done to rule out serious diseases, such as cancer, requiring appropriate primary therapy.

IMMUNE SYMPTOMS

The immune system consists of white blood cells as well as antibodies, bits of protein produced by the body to protect the body from "foreign" materials such as bacteria, etc. Immune disorders are most perplexing to physicians and patients. There is no specific diagnostic test for most immune diseases, and none of the subdiagnostic tests (such as Epstein-Barr virus titers) give proof of the clinically suspected diagnosis. In my experience, treatment with anticandida drugs gives only transient improvement, if any at all. Various allergy treatments are similarly ineffective. And of course, there is a wide variety of autoimmune diseases, in which the body mistakenly attacks itself. Rheumatoid arthritis and multiple sclerosis are examples of autoimmune diseases.

DEPRESSION

In many individuals, a major life crisis initiates a progressive disease. Often the crisis is enough at least to create a situational depressive reaction. Some of these individuals have a lifelong feeling of never having been happy. Occasionally the onset of the illness is an apparent viral infection, such as influenza, with slow and incomplete recovery and feelings of debilitation and depression, primarily because of radical life changes induced by the change in energy, work capacity, relationships, and so forth. Without depression demonstrable on the MMPI if not on the **Zung Self-Assessment Scale for Depression,** the diagnosis of EMD is not possible.

THIRTY OR MORE SYMPTOMS

The Cornell Medical Index (CMI) was touted a generation ago as adequate for making a clinical diagnosis with 80 percent accuracy, without physical examination or lab tests. The CMI included a family history and past history. If we take just symptoms, currently or within the past year, a finding of thirty or more symptoms means severe sympathetic overactivity, indicative of, at least, maladaptation. On the other hand, thirty or more symptoms might be present in serious illnesses such as cancer or psychosis. As with any problem, careful diagnostic testing must be done to rule out other treatable illnesses.

DHEA DEFICIENCY

Although much of the literature states that true DHEA deficiency, or adrenoandrogen deficiency, is diagnosable at less than 180 mg/dL in men or less than 130 mg/dL in women, DHEA levels below the mean (510 ng/dL in women; 715 ng/dL in men) imply progressively less adrenal reserve. All patients with EMD will have levels less than 50 percent of the mean, and none have levels at the mean or above. Relative DHEA deficiency is common and present in virtually every major illness as well as in chronic stress. The levels in EMD are not in themselves diagnostic, but they do suggest relative adrenal exhaustion or adrenal maladaptation.

DEFICIENT INTRACELLULAR MAGNESIUM

Eighty percent of women and 70 percent of men do not eat even the recommended daily intake of magnesium. Thus, magnesium deficiency is rampant and associated with most chronic illnesses. A low intracellular magnesium is not diagnostic of any disease, but EMD is inevitably associated with such deficiency. Magnesium regulates membrane potential. This deficiency thus contributes considerably to the increased sensitivity of patients with EMD.

DEFICIENCY IN
ESSENTIAL AMINO ACIDS

Malnutrition is common in many chronic illnesses and particularly in patients with chronic depression. The essential amino acids are needed to produce most neurochemicals. Thus norepinephrine, serotonin, melatonin, beta endorphin, all of which are crucial neurochemicals essential for feeling energetic, cannot be properly balanced with deficiencies of the building blocks. Taurine is now considered an essential amino acid by many scientists, and taurine is deficient in 86 percent of patients with depression. Cells normally have a negative charge on the cell wall or membrane. This negative charge keeps the cell from "firing," or discharging, its energy unless properly stimulated. The double deficiency of magnesium and taurine is particularly crucial in evoking the hypersensitivity of patients with EMD. Because patients are deficient in both magnesium and taurine, they are especially weakened and susceptible, hypersensitive to almost any threat to their physical system. In other words, their nervous system, particularly, fires too easily. This leads to agitation and depression.

EEG BRAIN-MAP ABNORMALITIES

Asymmetry of EEG activity (especially in the right frontal lobe) has been reported in patients with depression. And, indeed, all four EEG abnormalities noted earlier have been seen in patients with chronic depression, even when chronic fatigue and immune dysfunction are not the primary complaints. "Simple" dysthymia is thus invariably part of the syndrome I am calling EMD. Perhaps there is a broad band of dysfunction ranging from mild to severe depression and, in the extreme, mild to the most severe form of neurasthenia, with corresponding increasing sensitivity to a variety of stimuli.

HYPOTHESES ABOUT ELECTROMAGNETIC DYSTHYMIA

EMD may be the foundation for many illnesses. The simplest form of EMD includes significant depression with the four EEG abnormalities described. These abnormalities are created or aggravated by deficiency of magnesium and usually taurine, and further aggravated by deficiency of tyrosine, phenylalanine, isoleucine, leucine, tryptophan, vitamins B_1, B_2, B_3, or B_6, or lithium.

As the ability to cope with increasing stress is lost, homeostasis becomes erratic, and DHEA begins to decrease. "Total stress" includes nicotine, excess sugar and caffeine, smog and pollution, artificially hydrogenated fat, poor nutrition, inadequate physical exercise, lack of natural light, poor quality of interior air, and psychosocial pressure.

In addition, electromagnetic "pollution" has increasingly contributed to stress. Remember that *electromagnetic* includes both electricity and the magnetic force electricity produces. This electromagnetic energy is measured in milligauss. The earth's magnetic field is approximately one-half gauss. Exposure to over 3 milligauss of electromagnetic pollution produces excessive free radicals, perhaps even more than poor nutrition. Fluorescent lights, multiple electrical appliances and devices, automobiles, airplanes, radio and TV waves, and radar bombard the human energy system daily and may provide major electromagnetic stress, which appears to lead to an ever-increasing incidence of depression and EMD. In view of the fact that TV, radio, and cellular phones may interfere with the ability of pilots to navigate airplanes, we are naive to ignore the impact of multiple electromagnetic influences on the human brain, which is much more sensitive than flight instruments!

When we accept depression and various stress illnesses as indicative of electromagnetic (psychoneuroimmunologic) overload, we are approaching a primary principle of Sir William Osler: that there is one common cause of illness. That cause is chemical, physical, emotional, and electromagnetic stress that affects the limbic system and hypothalamus, leading to loss of electrical homeostasis of the brain/mind. The primary illness in electromagnetic dysthymia manifests as depression, with or without multiple system disease.

Having described this syndrome, how does it fit clinically? We have previously reported that patients with chronic pain are virtually always depressed and have an average of 49 symptoms. At least 70 percent of chronic-pain patients and 100 percent of those with chronic depression are deficient in magnesium; 86 percent are deficient in taurine; 100 percent are deficient in one or more essential amino acids; all those who are chronically depressed present the four EEG abnormalities; all show DHEA levels below the mean; most have one or more symptoms involving allergies or immune dysfunction; virtually all have some degree of fatigue or loss of energy; and neurochemical abnormalities occur in 100 percent of chronically depressed patients. In some patients the dominant symptoms are chronic fatigue and various allergic hypersensitivities. In others, other major associated symptoms of disease dominate. They have in common four EEG abnormalities: low DHEA, magnesium, and essential amino acids; multiple symptoms; depression; and varying degrees of fatigue. Chronic fatigue syndrome is simply one extreme of EMD.

TREATMENT OF
ELECTROMAGNETIC DYSTHYMIA

Major stress-reduction techniques provide the foundation for treatment. These include photostimulation, education, music, biofeedback, guided imagery, and autogenic training. Magnesium replacement and amino-acid supplementation may also assist recovery. DHEA restoration is of considerable benefit, as is the Liss stimulator (TENS device), applied both transcranially and to the twelve acupuncture points called the Ring of Fire. Eighty-five percent of patients respond initially to two weeks of intensive multimodal treatment, and 70 percent improve long term.

How does EMD relate to the great diseases of "modern" society: heart disease, cancer, stroke, diabetes, and others? The basic relation, as I see it, is that EMD is a reaction to total life stress. If we consider EMD a manifestation of burnout or overload of the electromagnetic framework, the primary etiological factor being stress, then each of the other illnesses represents overload in the organ system most involved. Fear, anxiety, resentment, anger, guilt, and the ultimate emotional stress—depression—block life energy and cause electromagnetic energetic deprivation on or in an organ or region with the greatest unresolved emotional distress.

In every illness, at some point, the energetic drain overloads the **adrenal glands,** thus weakening the very organ that ordinarily counterbalances stress. Thus adrenal burnout, a prominent feature of EMD, is also a component of every major disease. As long as the body is capable of restoring homeostasis, major disease does not occur and DHEA levels remain reasonably adequate. As the adrenals fail, DHEA progressively declines, weakening the immune system and decreasing total life energy.

ACUPUNCTURE

The most subtle physiological expression of electromagnetism is that activated by acupuncture. There are many aspects of acupuncture, not the least of which is the "traditional" Chinese concept of five elements. The ancient Chinese philosophy is not significantly different from ancient Greek philosophy and probably the ancient philosophy of most cultures.

The human is seen as a microcosm of the macrocosm, which, in China, is called Tao, the harmonizing force of the universe. The Chinese see everything as a continuum from Yin to Yang and back again, with Yin and Yang representing opposite but complementary aspects that are constantly moving and combining with each other, producing all that comes to be. The Chinese believe in a universal energy, the essence of life, called chi or qi (in Japan called ki). Everything is a manifestation of chi, either at a subtle, invisible level or a physical, material level. The Chinese believe that this life force circulates through acupuncture channels to protect, nourish, and animate life. (When Marco Polo brought back ancient Chinese texts and these were translated into French, the Jesuit influence converted the concept of qi to spirit.)

The Chinese see the meridians as pathways along which chi circulates to twelve regular pathways, eight extra meridians, and several other points. Along these meridians are acupuncture points and, interestingly, almost all acupuncture points represent depressions in areas in fibrofascial spots between muscles and tendons. Most acupuncture points are tender, and the stronger the acupuncture point, the more tender it is; or the more out of balance that particular meridian, the more tender the points may be.

The principle of acupuncture is that of returning the person to a state of homeostasis. If some negative "side effects" or symptoms appear with acupuncture, these are seen as part of the general rebalancing.

Much scientific research in the past twenty-five years has documented remarkable physiological effects produced by stimulation of very specific acupuncture points. Dr. Joseph Helms has demonstrated that use of acupuncture energetics is statistically significant in reducing the symptoms of premenstrual syndrome (PMS), and I have demonstrated using acupuncture that this circuit called tchong mo raises sperm count strikingly in infertile men. Furthermore, on numerous occasions I have used acupuncture to start menstrual periods in women who had delayed onset of menses or to stop excessive and prolonged bleeding. Even a single acupuncture treatment has stopped a heavy three-week bleeding that showed no other signs of cessation prior to my acupuncture treatment.

ACUPUNCTURE AND
THE RINGS OF LIFE

I believe DHEA is the chemical manifestation of one's life energy, or qi reserve. This would reflect or substantiate the Chinese concept of the kidneys as the reservoir of one's inherited qi. My first idea to raise DHEA was to use natural progesterone, and I did indeed demonstrate unequivocally that natural progesterone will raise DHEA from 30 to 100 percent in most individuals, with an average increase of 60 percent. However, if one starts at 180 ng/dl or below, even a 100 percent increase will not bring the individual into the normal range.

I then asked the question, "What else can I do?" The answer I came up with was to stimulate the energetic acupuncture points that connect the kidneys with the gonads with the adrenals, the thyroid gland, and the pituitary through a "Window of the Sky" point. **"Window of the Sky points"** are those in Chinese cosmology that connect body/mind with the cosmos, or spirit. As mentioned earlier, I chose to call this circuit the Ring of Fire.

In traditional acupuncture there is no acupuncture point for the pituitary, and I chose the acupuncture point called Governing Vessel 20, which overlies the pineal gland, assuming that this might work since the pineal controls the pituitary.* Results were most

---

*I also used the acupuncture points for: Kidney 3 (bilateral), Conception Vessel 2, Conception Vessel 6, Bladder 22 (bilateral), Conception Vessel 18, Master of the Heart 6 (bilateral), Large Intestine 18 (bilateral), and Governing Vessel 20—chosen intuitively. The proof of the pudding is in the eating.

gratifying. When I stimulated these points with the gigafrequency device from the Ukraine, the DHEA increased, again averaging about 60 percent over baseline. Since the GigaTENS™ device (54 to 78 billion cycles per second) was not commercially available, I then tried the Liss TENS™, which has been on the market since 1975; when this was applied to the same acupuncture points, similar results ensued.

Continuing the DHEA studies, I next discovered that a combination of 2 grams of vitamin C, 1 gram of methylsulfonylmethane, 6 mg. of beta 1, 3 glucan, and 60 mcg. of molybdenum also raised DHEA 60 to 100 percent. Each of these mechanisms appears to work somewhat differently, since a cumulative effect results when the four are added together. That is, there is an average increase of 60 percent in the DHEA level with each of them individually and an average of over 200 percent increase when all are used concomitantly.

The success was not limited to DHEA alone. Subsequent clinical experiences with the Ring of Fire have revealed that stimulation of the Ring of Fire with either the Liss TENS™ or the GigaTENS™ can reduce both the frequency and the severity of migraine headache by 75 percent in 76 percent of patients. In 80 percent of patients with diabetic neuropathy there is a marked reduction in pain, but this occurs only with the GigaTENS™ and not with the Liss stimulator. In 70 percent of rheumatoid arthritic patients I achieved a remarkable decrease in patients' pain level and an improved mobility, even in cases where prednisone, gold, and/or methotrexate treatments had not helped.

Later I introduced the use of the SheLi TENS™, as I found that it covers a wide variety of frequencies and has, among other frequencies, the same gigafrequency and intensity that is seen with the more specific Ukrainian devices—that is, by oscilloscopic monitoring, an output of 50 to 100 decibels of energy in the frequency from 54 to 78 gigahertz. This particular TENS is one that I have developed in the last four years and for which I have received FDA approval for manufacturing and sale. It is now available on physician prescription.

After my successes with the Ring of Fire, I began to perceive the presence of other energetic circuits within the human body. The second circuit was one that I chose to call the Ring of Air (note that the meridian points for the stimulations appear in chapter 2.)

Next I was intuitively guided to the Ring of Water. Interestingly, stimulation of the Ring of Water with the SheLi TENS™ moderately increased aldosterone, the hormone associated with water and mineral metabolism.

Next, I was intuitively given the Ring of Earth. Stimulation of the Ring of Earth with the SheLi TENS™ increased calcitonin levels quite strikingly.

Finally, I investigated a circuit called the Ring of Crystal. Stimulation of the Ring of Crystal with the Liss Stimulator or the SheLi TENS™ reduced free radicals over 90 percent in 86 percent of thirty patients tested to date.

It is my belief that ongoing electrical activation of at least the Ring of Fire, Ring of Earth, and Ring of Crystal points has the potential to rejuvenate life energy on a very broad scale, and, incredibly, to possibly regenerate the spinal cord. I have tried this in only two individuals. First was a forty-four-year-old man who had been paralyzed from L2 (location of a vertebra on the spinal column above the sacrum) down for some two years. After two and a half months of stimulation of the Ring of Crystal, he had achieved an orgasm for the first time, and his flaccid feet had begun to have very constant fine-motor fasciculations. Unfortunately, his fundamentalist religious beliefs led him to discontinue the process at that time. More recently, a forty-eight-year-old physician who is moderately quadriparetic started using the Ring of Crystal and the Ring of Earth and has achieved in a six-month period what he assesses as between 25 and 30 percent improvement in strength and motion in his shoulders and left leg. Many more studies need to be done with much longer follow-up, as I think it could take as long as seven years to regenerate the spinal cord.

In summary, throughout at least four thousand years philosophers have theorized not only that there is an energy that we call soul or spirit, but also that there is a universal energy that circulates throughout our environment that is necessary for life. In addition, theories have suggested that living beings not only absorb this energy but also circulate it in specific pathways inside the human body. Approximately 20 percent of individuals see a manifestation of the energy reflected around the human body as an "aura," and a much smaller percentage, perhaps one in one hundred thousand, see many more subtle aspects of this reflection of the body's internal energy.

Finally, through the use of acupuncture and specific types of electrical stimulation applied to the surface of the body, especially to acupuncture points, we appear capable of modulating a wide variety of neurochemicals, including serotonin, beta endorphin, DHEA, neurotensin, aldosterone, calcitonin, and free radicals. Future work will undoubtedly further refine these concepts of internal and external human energy.

RECOMMENDED READING ON ACUPUNCTURE

H. Beinfield and E. Korngold, *Between Heaven and Earth* (New York: Ballantine Books, 1991).

T. Kaptchuk, *Chinese Medicine: The Web That Has No Weaver* (New York: McGraw-Hill, 2000).

L. Hammer, *Dragon Rises, Red Bird Flies* (New York: Barrytown/Station Hill, 1990).

X. Cheng, *Chinese Acupuncture and Moxibustion* (Beijing: Foreign Language Press, 1987).

A. Ellis, N. Wiseman, and K. Boss, *Fundamentals of Chinese Acupuncture* (Brookline, Mass.: Paradigm Publications, 1988).

L. Yanchi, *The Essential Book of Traditional Chinese Medicine* (New York: Columbia University Press, 1988).

P. Deadman and M. Al-Khafaji, *A Manual of Acupuncture* (East Sussex, England: Journal of Chinese Medicine Publication, 1998).

J. M. Helms, *Acupuncture Energetics: A Clinical Approach for Physicians* (Berkeley, Calif.: Medical Acupuncture Publishers, 1995).

M. Sankey, ed., *Esoteric Acupuncture, Gateway to Expanded Healing* (Los Angeles: Mountain Castle Publishing, 1991).

F. Mann, *The Treatment of Disease by Acupuncture*, 2nd ed. (London: William Heinemann Medical Books Ltd., 1971).

F. Mann, *Scientific Aspects of Acupuncture* (London: William Heinemann Medical Books, 1977).

SUBTLE PHYSICAL ENERGETICS

As a scientist of life, one of the great questions for me is the connection between electromagnetism and the physical matter of life. Here we encounter the microscopic world, along with the work of several physicians who independently reported a variety of phenomena. This work was rejected by the medical establishment, just as electricity was originally rejected.

Royal Rife, Wilhelm Reich, Virginia Livingston, Günther Enderlein, Robert Koch, and Gaston Naessens all have emphasized the importance of minute, apparently "living" particles that may be the physical equivalent of "energy." Reich described small, moving, brightly reflective particles seen in the atmosphere. These are readily visible looking up into a blue sky on a bright sunny day. Reich believed these represented **orgone** itself. He went further and stated that similar "organisms" appeared in water, into which he placed a lump of coal.[96] These particular moving bright objects appearing *de nouveau* could be seen with a dark-field microscope.

Over sixty years later, scientists have reported that they "revived" twenty-five-year-old bacteria extracted from amber.[97] Similarly, I have extracted the "universal basic living material" from a fly in amber! My findings on the organisms studied are similar to those reported by Livingston and Naessens. Over a period of four years, I observed some of the characteristics of physically kinetic microscopic reflective particles or cells in animal and human blood and in various plant juices. These physically active cells have been studied under a variety of conditions at 1,000 magnification in a dark-field microscope. For want of a specific name, I will call them **L-cells**, for **life cells**.

THE HUMAN ENERGY FIELD

The term *human energy field* raises questions that have largely been ignored by conventional science and medicine. Although there was widespread use of electrical current in the 1700s, it was Abraham Flexner who denounced the use of electrical shocks in current, and it was Flexner's report that "drove all mention of it from the classroom and clinic." At the same time, the whole belief of "vital electricity" was purged from biology by the discovery of acetylcholine. Thus, medicine entered the chemical and biochemical field and gave electricity and electromagnetism a very secondary role. In the meantime, outside the field of biology, electricity changed the entire future of the world!

A few researchers plodded along, and perhaps the most significant of these was Harold Saxton Burr of Yale, who published most of his work in the *Yale Journal of Biology and Medicine*. Fortunately his book on the subject has been printed: *Blueprint for Immortality: The Electric Patterns of Light*.[98] Despite the paucity of elegant equipment, Burr and his co-workers found electric fields on the surfaces of organisms from worms and slime molds up through mammals and humans and, in fact, found electric fields around all living subjects. They correlated changes in potentials with "growth regeneration," tumor formation, drug effects, hypnosis, and sleep. They even demonstrated that trees respond not only to light and moisture but also to storms, sunspots, and phases of the moon. Burr called the electric field around an organism the "field of light" or the L-field. He stated, "When we meet a friend we have not seen for six months there is not one molecule in his face that was there when we last saw him. But thanks to his controlling L-field, the new molecules have fallen into the old familial pattern that we recognize and we can recognize his face."[99] Burr believed that abnormalities in the L-field could reveal latent illness and could predict a person's emotional and physical health, both past and present.

THE HUMAN AURA AND
THE ETHERIC BODY

This very brief introduction to the concept of energy fields and its possible implications in therapy would, of course, be fairly incomplete if I did not mention the ancient philosophical concept of the human aura and the theosophical concept of the **etheric body.** In 1927 Charles Leadbeater described the etheric body as "the vehicle through which flow the streams of vitality which keep the body alive, and [unless] it has a bridge to convey undulations of thought and feeling from the astral to the visible denser physical matter, the ego could make no use of the cells of [the] brain."[100] He goes on to state that "it is clearly visible to declare the clairvoyant as a mass of faintly-luminous violet-grey mist interpenetrating the denser part of the body, and extending very slightly beyond it."[101]

It has been my impression that approximately 20 percent of individuals see the etheric energy around the human body. A much smaller percentage see in that etheric energy various rotating wheel-shaped energy centers called "chakras." I have always seen what I call an energy field or an electromagnetic field around human beings. In general, it looks very much like heat waves rising off the pavement or off the hood of a car, although there are frequent, various and sundry colors in this energy field. In addition, around psychotic individuals I see a remarkable turbulence of energy that is often dark and very chaotic-looking, almost like a tornado, usually occurring around the right side of the head and shoulder. Interestingly, the late Dr. John Pierrakos, the most prominent student of Wilhelm Reich, described similar disruptions of energy around psychotics with a wide variety of patterns, depending upon the nature of the major psychological disorder.

When I first heard of the **chakras,** this made great sense to me because the six lower chakras overlie specific collections of nerve cells and plexi. Indeed, when one sees a schematic sketch of the nervous system as shown by Dr. Irvin Korr, these circuits virtually overlie the regions of the lower six chakras.[102] Only the seventh chakra, which is at the top of the head pointing upward, is not so specific, although one could consider it the upward projection from the brain itself. It is my impression that the first chakra is the representation of the sciatic plexus, the second the pelvic plexus, the fifth the cervical plexus, and the sixth the brain itself, although in the theosophical philosophy and its foundation, Eastern Indian philosophy, each of these chakras is more specifically related to glandular function.

LIFE AND COSMIC ENERGY

The question of how many dimensions exist in the universe is sometimes raised by scientists or others. We easily know about four dimensions: height, weight, depth, and time. But what about the fifth dimension? Let us assume that the difference in dimensions is ultimately frequency. At the level of the fifth dimension, neutrinos (similar to electrons but they do not carry an electric charge) represent one critical aspect of frequency, and an isotron represents the interdimensional change agent.

In the fourth dimension, sound and light are the primary manifestations. Ultimately light varies in frequency through the known electromagnetic range. Interactions of light, sound, and isotrons in the range of 40 to 80 GHz produce life as we know it. The simplest form of such life is the somatid. As complexity increases, the L-cells "become" various forms of microorganisms and ultimately become human beings. L-cells represent the essential life energy, chi, prana, or the *living* erg.

In the fifth dimension, the frequency is so high that there is no time or space; everything coexists. Only the mind can transcend dimensions perfectly from the fourth to the fifth dimension. When the mind transcends perfectly into the fifth dimension, it perceives, or "knows," everything that is; it is then able to *direct* ultimate energy to create matter (materialize), disintegrate matter (dematerialize) or heal, or bring into realization (manifest) ideas from the *ultimate Source*.

Physical manifestation, whether nonliving or living, represents the most compacted form of energy. Only when this energy is regulated by a *specific* fourth-dimensional cybernetic energy is life infused into this compacted physical energy. Water is essential for the survival of this basic life energy, the L-cell described earlier. Water is the interfacing physical/etheric energy that allows isotron transformation into life.

The cybernetic fifth-dimensional energy that directly "creates" human life is the soul. That is, the soul is the transducer of life from the fifth dimension. However, there may be other fifth-dimensional cybernetic transducers for the life force for plants and animals.

More complex cybernetic energy is responsible for evolution of the soul (and all of creation). This includes angels, archangels, and ultimately, the most complex energy: the Force, or God.

Since life is a compaction (condensation) of light, it is dependent upon all aspects of the visible spectrum for sustenance. In order to optimize the input of light (color), there are specific energy receptacles, subtransducers, or chakras that transform color into energy regulation/modulation. Metaphysically, many philosophers and intuitives have suggested that there are levels of life energy beyond the visible spectrum. The etheric "body" is the first level of energy outside the physical body and thought by many to be the connecting energetic system between soul and body. Then in concentric layers outside the etheric body there are the astral, or emotional, body; the mental body; the causal body, etc. The "aura" seen by many appears to be a subtle energy that may be etheric or a combination of etheric and astral energy. Certainly, much of what I see appears to be influenced by the mental/emotional state of the person. Major metaphysical questions concerning these states of energy remain outside current science. Perhaps when we truly understand the electromagnetic aspects of life, L-cells, etc., the physics of these presumed aspects of life will begin to be studied. Even the concept of thought forms is not well understood. But the effect of thought has been demonstrated well in my experiments with five healers who, in 116 individuals, have been able to alter the EEG from distances up to 1,000 miles. Thought forms, called the "collective unconscious" by Carl Jung, represent fourth-dimensional influences of massive cumulative human emotions. There are universal archetypal patterns that were introduced in the writings of Jung. Mother, father, child, victim, etc., are concepts that have universal meaning and energetic influences in society as well as in individuals. Caroline Myss has taken these concepts much further in her magnificent book *Sacred Contracts*. Her concept that we are born to learn to use power wisely, responsibly, and lovingly is most appealing. And those who work with the "contracts" find them to be powerful tools for insight, and ultimately, therapy.

The chakras represent the Energetic Regulating System for the electrical core battery of the body, the *Ring of Fire*. This core consists of the coherent energy system K 3, CV 2, B 22, CV 6, CV 18, MH 6, LI 18, GV 20 (key acupuncture points), the flow of energy from pituitary to Window of the Sky to thyroid, master of the heart, adrenals, gonads, kidneys, and uterus or prostate. The most sensitive acupuncture point for the first chakra is K 3; the second, CV 2 and CV 6; the third, B 22; the fourth, MH 6; the fifth, LI 18; and the sixth and seventh share GV 20. Obviously many related points may also influence the Ring of Fire or specific organs.

When stress is greater than the Ring of Fire can sustain, life-energy intensity and/or frequency are reduced, and the Ring of Fire's regulation of the other energy pathways (meridians) begins to become inadequate. As this happens, glandular regulation also becomes inefficient. Cholesterol then cannot be converted into DHEA adequately and may build up in the blood or be deposited in arteries. The DHEA level decreases, but other hormones remain within "normal" limits (testosterone, estrogen, thyroid, aldosterone, and various pituitary hormones). When the DHEA level falls below the essential level for health, increasing energy deficits eventually lead to gross electrical dysfunction (reflected in the EKG, EEG, cell membrane potential, etc.), then chemical dysfunction, and finally physical damage or illness.

Anything that reduces stress adequately may allow the natural homeostatic nature of the Ring of Fire to be restored. All forms of relaxation, sound, light, music, and mental peacefulness may assist this process. With the cooperation of the mind, electricity (TENS applied transcranially), quartz crystals, homeopathy, nutrition, and millimeter waves (called Magnetic Resonance Therapy, or MRT, in the Ukraine, but I prefer the name GigaTENS™) may assist in the restoration of the Ring of Fire and subsequent healing. Spiritual healing may influence the Ring of Fire directly by transmitting fourth-dimensional energy into the chakras from the major personal transducer, the soul.

STRESS INFLUENCES

- Obviously, at a physical level, chemical and physical interventions may also assist in restoration of chemical and/or physical balance. Acupuncture probably affects the human energy system by serving as an antenna for collecting solar millimeter waves.
- Massage and postural adjustments may serve as physical enhancers or by transfer (focusing) of electromagnetic and/or millimeter waves.
- Barometric pressure affects various electromagnetic and cosmic energetics. Astrological influences occur through gravitational, electromagnetic, and cosmic (fourth-dimensional or eighth chakra) energetics.
- Specific emotional stress may deprive specific chakras of their life-sustaining energy. For instance: fear related to all aspects of physical safety, family, or "rootedness," may affect the first chakra; fear related to sexuality

and/or financial security affects the second chakra; fear of relationships, responsibility, and self-worth affects the third chakra; fear of love (abandonment/abuse and subsequent anger, hatred, judgmentalism) affects the fourth chakra; fear of expression of personal needs or desires (will) affects the fifth chakra; fear related to "knowing," intuition, and/or wisdom affects the sixth chakra; and fear of existence (purpose, meaning) affects the seventh chakra.

The differential reaction to fear depends upon the intensity/quality of the fear and its reaction in the form of anxiety, guilt, anger, or depression. Additionally, the combination of fears related to all seven chakras influences the specific illness, which may manifest from continuing chakra overload, deprivation, or blockage. When fear is unresolved, there is a *reverse* energy loss or transfer of incoming energy, which continues draining (blocking) the appropriate chakra until either the fear is totally resolved or physical illness ensues.

When the seventh chakra is drained (blocked), there is a generalized energetic shortage for all the chakras. The specific illnesses developing depend upon the combination of energetic depletion in a given chakra, as well as the shortfall from the seventh chakra.

Emotional unfinished business (fear) resulting in guilt, anxiety, or depression prevents the mind from attuning to the eighth chakra or higher.

Energetic imbalances may include excesses or deficiencies because of blocks and short circuits in the natural flow or vector-potentials (meridians) from the organs.

In health, the soul transforms cosmic energy into the seventh chakra, and the energy flows in an organized pattern through the body, restoring and rejuvenating it. Balance is achieved by releasing excess accumulated energy through orgasm or through creativity (transforming receiving ideas into physical manifestation). When creativity is blocked, obesity may result or depression may occur. When orgasm is denied, then energy may accumulate in the second chakra or any other system to which it is transmitted through magnetic attraction or by short-circuiting. Orgasm is one energetic technique for establishing coherence or balance in the Ring of Fire and meridian system. Meditation, when optimally performed, may also lead to such coherence.

Mindfulness/focus/grounding in the now/present also assists this process of coherence. When all attachment to past trauma (fear) is resolved, the system is optimally coherent.

Although this concept of electromagnetism and cosmic energy may seem complicated in considering health and well-being, once again we have the simple fact that everything affects everything. Ultimately there is a universal power, usually called God. Every known physical, chemical, electrical, magnetic, mental, and emotional energy interacts to determine ultimate balance—or health.

Throughout history philosophers and mystics have reflected upon the energy of life. In every culture, except modern scientific monotheism, life is considered sacred, the physical manifestation of spiritual energy emanating from a divine source, God. Ninety percent of Americans share a common belief in God and in life after death (the soul). But science has ignored or suppressed interest in the spiritual nature of life itself since the days of Descartes' famous statement "I think, therefore I am."

Even the concept of thinking, poorly understood by scientists, religious leaders, and laypersons, defies scientific explanation. In their attempt to make humans the ultimate creation, many scientists have insisted that other animals don't think, plan, play, or have emotions. How ignorant! (Incidentally, ignorance, as Edward Bach has defined it, is simply the failure to accept truth.) Thinking is one aspect of life, but not the only one. As Antonio Damasio has elegantly explained in *Looking for Spinoza: Joy, Sorrow, and the Feeling Brain*, emotions are the body's sensations that must be *felt* with the conscious, thinking, and ultimately "feeling" brain.[103]

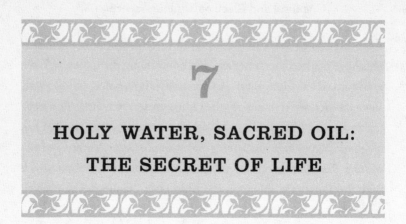

7

HOLY WATER, SACRED OIL: THE SECRET OF LIFE

WATER, WATER EVERYWHERE AND NOT A DROP TO DRINK

From a scientific point of view, the most essential factor for human life is air and the second is water. We can live without air for approximately three minutes. Depending on the air temperature, we can live without water for up to two weeks. The human body is composed of a minimum of 70 percent water, and virtually every living process requires water for the chemical events essential to life. Water enables us to maintain our normal body temperature. We carry waste products out of the body through water. For the last 100 years, physicians have recommended that the average adult consume about two quarts of water per day.

But what about the quality of water? West of Missouri, almost all water is relatively "soft," for its alkali content. East of the Missouri–Kansas line, almost all water is "hard," containing calcium and magnesium. Deaths from heart disease are lower in areas where the drinking water is hard. Artificially softened water, which is often used in the hard-water areas, is extremely unsafe, as the calcium and magnesium are often replaced with sodium, and the zinc in the pipelines may be replaced with cadmium. Cadmium is leached out of pipes by the sodium used to replace magnesium and calcium removed from hard water.[104] More important, over the last seventy-five years the vast majority of municipal water has been chlorinated and fluoridated, the latter theoretically just to prevent dental decay. And yet there is no benefit of fluoride after age seven, and it may create fragile bones.[105] There is increasing evidence that chlorine may be more harmful than sodium. Certainly we do not need extra chlorine in our bodies. Furthermore, chlorine interferes with absorption of iodine, which, in my opinion, is partly responsible for relatively common subclinical hypothyroidism.

One of the other problems with chlorination of water is that if there is any contamination of the municipal water with any byproducts of sewage, the chlorine may convert these into carcinogenic agents. About every ten years a little blurb gets out into the national media about the fact that chlorinated water contains carcinogens. But there is no way for city water to be provided safely without chlorination because the chlorination is added specifically to kill those bacteria that come from sewage contamination! In other words, we have to chlorinate the water to prevent bacterial infection, but somehow we have to get rid of the chlorine to make it truly healthy.

Even more worrisome is that for the last sixty years most cities have fluoridated their water. There is increasing evidence that fluoride is particularly harmful to bones; when used over a lifetime it may aggravate osteoporosis and cause the bones to become more brittle.[106] Distilled water has no minerals in it, and drinking two quarts of distilled water a day could leach some of the normal minerals from your body.

The best source of water is spring water or groundwater that has been carefully tested to be certain that it has not been contaminated with petrochemicals or bacteria. Those lucky individuals who have access to their own well and groundwater should have the water tested for contamination at least every three to five years. The place to do that is the Water Test Corporation, P.O. Box 6360, Manchester, NH 03108-6360 (phone 1-800-426-8378). Your local health department will analyze the water for bacterial contamination.

DEHYDRATION AS THE CAUSE OF ILLNESS—DR. F. BATMANGHELIDJ'S THEORIES ON WATER

In 1992, F. Batmanghelidj published an interesting medical commentary on water, titled *Your Body's Many Cries for Water*.[107] Dr. Batmanghelidj says unequivocally, "It is chronic dehydration that is the root cause of many of the diseases we confront in medicine at the present!" Batmanghelidj, born in Iran in the 1930s, has long been an advocate of the healing power of water. He believes that there is no substitute for water—not tea, coffee, alcohol, juice, or any other manufactured beverage. He says that he has treated over three thousand peptic ulcer sufferers *with water alone*. He believes that "dry mouth" is a symptom only at the "end stages" of dehydration and that this dehydration is responsible for dyspepsia or heartburn, rheumatoid pain, back pain, anginal pain, headache, leg pain, and indeed, most illnesses.

The doctor tells of a young man in his twenties who came to see him one evening in excruciating pain. The patient had taken cimetidine, 300 milligrams, as well as a full bottle of antacids, which had not relieved his heartburn pain. Dr. Batmanghelidj prescribed one pint of water, then fifteen minutes later one-half pint of water. Within twenty minutes the man's pain had totally disappeared. Dr. Batmanghelidj believes that in less severe cases, simple water will relieve gastric duodenal pain totally within eight minutes. He goes further to say that pain of colitis, or colon pain or "false appendicitis pain," is also equally relieved by adequate intake of water.

Although one might easily understand that water would dilute the excess acid (one of the foundations for gastric pain), it is perhaps more difficult to see how this could affect many other diseases. Dr. Batmanghelidj feels that simple, essential hypertension is a "gross body water deficiency signal." We know that in hypertension the peripheral blood vessels constrict. Dr. Batmanghelidj believes that the constriction is due to a loss of blood volume. In addition, he also feels that high blood cholesterol is the result of the body protecting itself. The cholesterol becomes something of a sludge to prevent the cells from further dehydrating. When one drinks adequate water, the cholesterol isn't needed to protect against dehydration and the cholesterol level will go down.

In the case of rheumatoid arthritis, he explains that the actively growing blood cells in bone marrow take priority over cartilage for available water. If a person is relatively dehydrated, then the bone marrow gets the fluid and the cartilage suffers. He therefore believes that joint pain is due to dehydration of the cartilage and subsequent inflammation.

Even allergies and asthma, he believes, are symptoms of dehydration. He argues that when a person is dehydrated, more histamine is produced to cause constriction of the bronchial muscle so that less water is lost through the lungs. As one becomes more and more dehydrated, more histamine is produced. He states that with adequate water intake, histamine production will decrease over a period of three to four weeks and bring the unique symptoms of allergies and asthma under control.

Dr. Batmanghelidj argues that anxiety and depression are also the results of water deficiency. Water is necessary for the chemical production of electricity in our brains. When we are relatively dehydrated, the level of energy generation is decreased. When there is inadequate energy production, we become depressed or irritable, which also means anxious.

Migraine headaches affect some 17 percent of women and 9 percent of men in this country. According to Dr. Batmanghelidj, migraine headaches are brought about by dehydration. He states that "the most prudent way of dealing with migraine is its prevention by the regular intake of water."

Finally, Dr. Batmanghelidj argues that water can also cure one of the most insidious diseases in America today, obesity. He describes two individuals who lost between thirty and forty-five pounds and another who lost fifty-eight pounds by only drinking water without diet change. He recommends always drinking a full glass of water thirty minutes before a meal and at least that much two and half hours after a meal, then two more glasses of water "around the heaviest meal or before going to bed"—a daily total of eight glasses, eight ounces each. Dr. Batmanghelidj makes the very important observation that if we eat food when we are dehydrated, the concentrated digestive products "draw water" from the cells. Indeed, this is, in my opinion, one of his most important points.

Research needs to be done to determine whether Dr. Batmanghelidj's concepts are correct. If they are, and I believe he is correct, it appears that we could solve many of America's medical problems if everyone drank two quarts of water a day. But remember, it must be nonchlorinated water and not coffee, tea, juice, or alcohol.

HEALING SPRINGS

From the late 1800s to the 1940s, the popularity of healing springs all over the world peaked. Medical professionals of the time were great proponents of water cures. Spas around the world enjoyed thousand of visitors, drawn to the hot springs by promises of health, cure, and overall well-being. One such spot is Excelsior Springs in Missouri, which is home to several different springs. In fact, the town boasts sixteen separate wells in the area, with water coming from as shallow as 10 feet, and as deep as 1,460 feet.[108] Some produce carbonated **ferro-manganese waters** that are believed to increase hemoglobin, temperature, pulse, and weight. They also increase appetite and reduce intestinal activity. Maybe it was acceptable in 1940, but I would not recommend this one!

Sulphato-carbonate waters are rich in calcium bicarbonate and are especially helpful in cases of obstinate chronic diarrhea. Uric acid, gravel (granules like sand), and calculi (stones) are also disintegrated and eliminated by the free use of this class of water.

Chloro-carbonate waters, better known as soda wells, are heavily charged with sodium chloride and bicarbonate combination. They are said to increase the health of the skin when applied externally. Although there are no scientific studies proving absorption of this water, it is theoretically believed by enthusiasts that these spring waters act as a tonic internally to correct acidity, increase the flow of gastric juice, improve appetite, increase the flow of urine and excretion of urea, and prevent putrefactive changes in the intestines.

In the 1940s, my mother visited Hot Springs every year. I accompanied her a few times and saw many individuals who swore the baths had cured them. In general, hot soaks, even at home, with magnesium chloride added to the water, are both detoxifying and rejuvenating. I take them at least five times a week in spring, fall, and winter and once or twice each week in the summer.

Chloride waters are said to carry the highest percentage of sodium chloride recorded in any of the Excelsior Spring waters. They often act as purgatives. The sulphato-chloride waters are especially indicated for catarrhal conditions of the mucous membranes of the stomach, intestines, and biliary passages as well as the urinary tract. They increase the flow of urine and the excretion of uric acid. In large quantities they act as purgatives.

Another well-known spring is found at the St. Moritz, Switzerland, health spa. Located at an altitude of 1,800 meters above sea level in a broad valley opening up toward the southwest, it offers a strongly stimulating Alpine climate that has dry air and is low in allergens. The mineral sources at St. Moritz are considered the strongest iron sources with carbonic acid in Europe. It is said that taking mineral baths at St. Moritz leads to a strong dilatation of blood vessels, thereby resulting in an intensification of blood circulation, reduction of high blood pressure, and a general vivifying and refreshing effect. It is also believed to be useful for treating the aftereffects of myocardial infarction (heart attack).

The chalybeate (iron-containing) water of the mineral source also contains many precious trace elements. It is said to stimulate digestion, kidney activity, and hematopoiesis (formation/development of blood cells). At the spa, peat baths and packs are used for treating chronic degenerative and inflammatory diseases, rheumatic disease, peritonitis, menstrual troubles, and for stimulating the adrenals and ovaries. Spa enthusiasts believe that these applications increase estrogen in the blood.

Lourdes is the best-known holy spring in the modern world. Bernadette Soubirous, a young, poor, and uneducated French girl, began having visions of the Virgin Mary. When she had one of these visions, she went into a state of "ecstasy." On February 25, 1858, Bernadette was praying at a grotto called Massabielle. Her fame had grown to the point that many people came to see her. She turned from the grotto and started toward the nearby river, then she turned back to the grotto and began digging in the dirt. A muddy ooze seeped from the hole and Bernadette attempted to drink it, but soon very clear water began to trickle from this spot toward the river. (The water flows today at a rate of over thirty thousand gallons a day.) People began to imitate Bernadette and to drink and wash with the water. As sick individuals got well and the injured became cured, the water began to be called miraculous.

By 1981 only sixty-five cases examined at Lourdes were declared by the Catholic Church to be miraculous, and millions of people worldwide have claimed that they have been cured or helped by the water of this spring. The water from the spring has been piped to taps and baths at the grotto and is bottled and shipped all over the world.

WEATHER, WATER, AND HEALTH

Hippocrates, the "father of medicine," emphasized the importance of climate and the seasons on health and disease. He wrote extensively about the influence of weather, especially heat and cold and water:

> All diseases occur at all seasons, but some diseases are more apt to occur and to be aggravated at certain seasons. . . . It is chiefly the changes of the seasons which produce diseases, and in the seasons the great changes from cold or heat, and so on according to the same rule.[109]

> For knowing the changes of the seasons, the rising and setting of the stars, how each of them takes place, he will be able to know beforehand what sort of a year is going to ensue. . . . and if it shall be thought that these things belong rather to meteorology, it will be admitted, on second thoughts, that astronomy contributes not a little, but a very great deal, indeed to medicine for with the seasons the digestive organs of men undergo a change.[110]

Modern research reveals that the most definitive aspects of weather are temperature, relative humidity, and barometric pressure. All these affect the relative hydration of the body, or the body's water balance. Rising temperature, falling humidity, and falling barometric pressure increase the number of health complaints and symptoms including:

- Fatigue
- Bad moods/depression/irritability

- Headaches
- Restless/disturbed sleep
- Poor concentration
- Nervousness
- Pain
- Emergency-room visits
- Increased mistakes
- Forgetfulness
- Dizziness
- Heart palpitations
- Psychotic breaks
- Higher blood pressure
- Delayed reaction times
- Death rate
- Suicides
- Birth/delivery rates
- Decrease in conception rates
- Colds
- Asthma
- Heart attacks
- Glaucoma
- Infections

Falling temperature, rising barometric pressure, and rising humidity improve health. About half of healthy people report being weather sensitive. Even healthy people who are not aware of being weather sensitive have increased symptoms during the weather risk conditions listed above. More critically, individuals who are already ill or weak have a markedly increased sensitivity to weather changes.

Weather changes are stressors that strongly influence health, illness, and death. These weather changes force biorhythms to high peaks and deep depressions.

Equally ignored but critically important are reactions to drugs. Individuals should carefully monitor themselves and **decrease dosages of these drugs during hot weather:**

Alcohol
Anticoagulants
Antihypertensives
Anti-Parkinson's drugs
Antispasmodics
Atropinelike drugs/belladonna
Cortisone/prednisone
Neuroleptics
Parasympathomimetics
Phenothiazines
Sedatives
Sleeping pills
Diuretics
All tranquilizers/tricyclic antidepressants

During cold weather the following drugs should be decreased:

Analgesics
Barbiturates
Hallucinogens
Monoamine oxidase inhibitors
Neuroleptics
Narcotics

Tetracyclines
All tranquilizers

How much? Obviously careful attention and medical caution should be foremost, but dosages might optimally be decreased 10 to 25 percent under extreme temperature changes. Alternatively, I believe that those adults who drink at least two quarts of water per day will maintain cell hydration better. And, of course, it seems probable that as the health of these individuals improves, their need for drugs will decrease.

IONS

Positive or negative ions in the air also affect us tremendously. Nature provides many ways to produce the more health-enhancing negative ions—rain; lightning; just clean, humid air. Hot, dry air and most air in buildings are more loaded with positive ions. Many air purifiers produce ozone, which, in small quantities, increases negative ions. As early as the 1930s, Swedish engineer Nils Lindebald noted that exposure to **positive polarity** led to depression and exposure to **negative polarity** led to striking improvements in mood. Viruses are repelled by negative ions and attracted to humans by positive ions. When the body becomes positive, viruses "attack" humans more powerfully.

Lindenbald and his supervisor, Dr. Clarence Hansell, chief of the RCA Radio Transmission Lab on Long Island, reasoned that there might be a link between man-made ions and those produced in nature, and they proved their hypothesis. They also learned that gas flames and electric heaters produced positive ions similar to those caused in this country by the Santa Ana winds. Students became more drowsy in a closed classroom, for example, probably because of the imbalance of light and the increase of positive ions produced by fluorescent lights. Lindebald and Hansell's research led to findings that high blood pressure could be treated without drugs by negative ionization of the atmosphere. Asthma was improved in 60 percent of asthmatics.[111] This is accomplished by negative ion generators, which are available from many sources. Search online and choose a reputable dealer.

Effects of positive ions include:

Fatigue

Headache

Dizziness

Nausea

Breathing difficulties

Asthma

Sinusitis

Pain, especially in arthritis

Increased blood pressure and pulse

Slower healing

More infections

Depression

Nervousness

Bad temper

Lack of confidence

Effects of negative ions include:

Optimism
Exhilaration
Good temper
Confidence
Relief of hay fever, asthma, sinusitis
Decreased blood pressure and pulse
Faster wound healing
Decreased pain
Decreased growth of transplanted cancer

In the late 1990s I was introduced to a variety of materials that altered water, possibly influencing hydrogen bonding and production of negative ions. These include **gold iodide crystals** and a micoid laminar crystal, each of which appears to have a different effect. Individuals who lie for twenty to thirty minutes on a bed of gold iodide crystals report going into very deep states of relaxation and awaken totally refreshed. It is as if they have had a complete release of tension in the body.

Lying on a bed of micoid laminar crystals, on the other hand, is quite energizing, and so it is almost impossible to fall asleep on that bed. Twenty to thirty minutes on the micoid laminar bed does an even better job of reenergizing the body and mind. I have worked with scores of individuals who consistently report the same benefits.

Micoid laminar crystal also affects water. When a hot tub is surrounded by six tons of the micoid laminar crystal, the water seems to be much softer, and individuals who have been in this crystal chamber feel significantly energized by the experience. The water, which has been conditioned by the micoid laminar crystals, tastes much softer than other water, and individuals report feeling as if it has a beneficial health effect. Many anecdotal reports of improved health have been received from individuals from soaking in the crystal-enhanced water and drinking this water. And grass seeds grown in this water sprout 20 percent more growth in the first week.

Results from my own experiments using water energized by the micoid laminar crystal are also quite striking. Grass seed, which has been watered with this particular energized water, grows much faster and thicker than a similar amount of grass seed watered without the micoid laminar energy. After one week, the grass seed fed by the micoid-laminar crystal water has a weight 20 percent greater than that watered with regular water.

Finally, I have constructed a quartz crystal room, the Rejuva-Matrix ™, eight by ten feet, and eight feet high, in which the walls and ceiling are made of quartz crystal, one ton in all. Most individuals go into a very deep state of rest and relaxation within moments of entering the crystal room and come out after thirty minutes totally rejuvenated. Those who experience the "crystal spa" for three to five days feel totally rejuvenated.

MY INITIAL MEASUREMENTS OF THE ACUPUNCTURE meridians, measured with the Asyra®, also show definite improvements in energy balance. The Asyra, an electronic device for measuring the electrical balance of the acupuncture meridians, is one of my favorite scientific tools for measuring efficacy of an energetic intervention. The gold iodide and micoid crystal beds and the crystal-enhanced hot tub/spa are often the beginning of a process that can be continued at home by soaking at least several times a week in a tub with the crystal-enhanced magnesium chloride solution. (When one mixes magnesium chloride in pure water, it produces a material that feels and looks like a thin oil.)

The secret of life appears to be replacement of magnesium, reenergizing and rebuilding of cells using electrical stimulation with DNA frequencies (using the SheLi TENS™), experiencing the crystal spa, and regularly using crystal-enhanced magnesium-chloride soaks. This may be the secret to achieving the longevity that people have been looking for so many years! This combination may indeed be the Secret of the Fountain of Youth!

RECOMMENDATIONS FOR EVERYONE
- Minimum of three soaks each week with one or two cups of the magnesium-chloride crystals.
- Use of the SheLi TENS™ on the Rings of Fire, Air, and Crystal, at least once each week

OPTIMAL JUMP-START
FOR THOSE WITH BURNOUT
- Three to five days of initial rejuvenation with gold-iodide and micoid-crystal beds, the crystal-enhanced spa, and the RejuvaMatrix quartz crystal room.

Performing this jump-start, individuals can speed the process tremendously. But even consistent use of the Recommendations for Everyone will accomplish great improvement over the first year. I have been doing this for three years now, and many comment on how much younger I look. Also, it is the only way I can keep my free radicals at a healthy, low level.

8

RECOMMENDATIONS FOR OPTIMAL HEALTH

BASICS FOR EVERYONE

DIET

Emphasize fruits, vegetables, nuts, and a wide variety of flesh foods (fish, beef, chicken, pork, etc.)

Whole grains in moderation, and potatoes and starches in moderation

Butter (*never* margarine), olive oil, and coconut oil are the major added fats to be used.

One to two eggs daily, unless you have *familial* hyper-cholesterolemia

Old-fashioned peanut butter, *never* hydrogenated or with
   sugar (Smuckers® is best)
Cheese, yogurt, buttermilk, unless allergic to milk

SUPPLEMENTS
90 to 100 pounds:

   2 Dr. sHEALy's Essentials® tablets
   3 Dr. sHEALy's Youth Formula® tablets
   2 teaspoons Biogenics® Magnesium Lotion on skin twice
      daily

111 to 130 pounds:

   3 Dr. sHEALy's Essentials® tablets
   4 Dr. sHEALy's Youth Formula® tablets
   2 teaspoons Biogenics® Magnesium Lotion on skin twice
      daily

Above 130 pounds:

   4 Dr. sHEALy's Essentials® tablets
   4 Dr. sHEALy's Youth Formula® tablets
   3 teaspoons Biogenics® Magnesium Lotion on skin twice
      daily

ALL men after age fifty:

Beta sitosterol, 1,200 mg. daily

EXERCISE
At least three hours weekly of moderate activity. Optimal is seven to fourteen hours!

SELF-REGULATION
At least thirty minutes daily of deep relaxation, autogenic training, meditation, etc. Avoid negative news in depth, violent movies, TV, etc. Appreciate nature and the Divine! Best presented in my book *90 Days to Stress-Free Living*. Relax at least thirty minutes daily. We have found the Shealy RelaxMate II™ to be the best adjunct for relaxation if you cannot relax quickly and easily. Relaxation is the greatest antidote to stress. Daily relaxation for thirty minutes lowers adrenaline production and insulin requirements by 50 percent for twenty-four hours.

OUTSIDE
At least one hour daily

SEX
At least two to three times weekly. If you do not have a partner, learn to enjoy masturbation!

WATER
At least two quarts daily, nonchlorinated.

SPECIFIC PROBLEMS AND ALTERNATIVES

ATTENTION-DEFICIT/HYPERACTIVITY DISORDER (ADHD)

I believe this disorder is grossly overdiagnosed and that Ritalin should be reserved for those who fail to respond to the safe, conservative approach below. Furthermore, I think there is *never* an excuse for Prozac® in this situation. Instead, give:

- Lithium orotate, 5 to 45 mg. daily (5 mg. for 50 pounds, gradually increasing to 45 mg. for 150 pounds weight)
- Taurine, 1,000 to 3,000 mg. daily
- Biogenics® Magnesium Lotion, 2 teaspoons on skin once or twice daily
- Photostimulation with the RelaxMate one hour daily
- Biogenics® tapes—start with Basic Schultz Autogenic Training daily
- Avoid sugar, pop, carbonated soft drinks, and aspartame.
- EEG biofeedback is also very good but requires one or two sessions a week for six months. (I would recommend it only when the above is not effective.)

Finally, if all the above fail, I would use the SheLi TENS™ on the Rings of Air and Earth.

ALCOHOLISM/ADDICTION

Basics plus:

- Ring of Earth stimulation with SheLi TENS™, plus stimulation of the addiction points, bilaterally
- Lithium orotate, as above
- Follow the recommendations in my book *90 Days to Stress-Free Living*.

If not doing well within one month maximum, get past-life therapy.

ALLERGIES

Most allergies are at least aggravated by food allergies. Start by avoiding wheat, milk products, eggs, citrus, corn, and peanuts, the most common food problems.

ADD:

- Beta-carotene 100,000 to 200,000 units daily
- Dr. sHEALy's Youth Formula®, four daily—contains 2 grams vitamin C, 1 gram MSM, 6 mg. beta 1,3 glucan, and 60 mcg. molybdenum
- Vitamin E, 400 units
- Co-Q 10, 100 mg. daily

If more is needed, see "Enhancing Immune Function," below.

ALZHEIMER'S DISEASE

Obviously use all the Basics recommendations for everyone.

At the earliest signs, add the following:

- If DHEA is below 200 in a woman or 300 in a man add DHEA, 100 mg. daily, assuming that the PSA is normal.
- Lecithin granules, two heaping tablespoons twice daily
- Stimulation of Ring of Fire daily, *plus* alternate Ring of Air, Earth, and Crystal
- Vitamin B$_{12}$ at least 1,000 mcg. daily
- Co-Q 10, 400 mg. daily
- Folic acid, 100 mg. daily

ANXIETY/PANIC DISORDER
Add to Basics:

- Double the amount of Biogenics® Magnesium Lotion
- Read and practice *90 Days to Stress-Free Living* (book).
- Work up to two hours daily of exercise.
- Use the RelaxMate twenty minutes three times daily.

ASTHMA
Basics plus instructions above for "Anxiety/Panic Disorder" plus "DHEA Restoration."

Magnesium replacement is essential, especially use of Magnesium Lotion.

Consider food allergy as a contributor—avoid wheat, corn, milk products, eggs, and citrus for a month.

AUTOIMMUNE DISEASES *(Lupus, Rheumatoid Arthritis, Scleroderma, Ulcerative Colitis, etc.; see also Irritable Bowel/Crohn's)*
All the Basics plus "Enhancing Immune Function" approaches. The Rings are especially recommended, alternating days with Rings of Fire, Earth, and Crystal.

The Seuterman homeopathic approach ("Seuterman Homeopathy," below) has also been particularly helpful in scleroderma and rheumatoid arthritis. Contact me for a specific protocol (normshealy@normshealy.net).

Practice the techniques in my book *90 Days to Stress-Free Living.*

BRAIN CANCER
There are no "proven" alternatives, and chemotherapy may be even worse than in other cancers. There are anecdotal reports of cures of six brain tumors. For information, contact John Sewell, 327 Charity Road, Homer, GA, 30547; 706-677-4934.

CANCER, GENERAL
In general, I do not find most of the somewhat radical approaches to be helpful to many people.

In addition to the "Enhancing Immune Function" approaches (below), I do recommend:

- Intravenous vitamin C, 75 to 100 grams daily for two to four weeks. This needs to have with it 100 mg. vitamin B_6, 1 cc. B complex 100, 2 grams magnesium chloride, 1 gram calcium chloride, and 1 gram Dex-Panthenol, all in a liter of IV fluid.

I believe that the best diet is one or two meals a day of macrobiotic and the other one or two totally raw foods.

One patient cured herself of metastatic cancer to the liver by using abdominal castor-oil packs and each night packing the soles of her feet with crushed raw garlic about one cm. thick, putting on socks, and continuing until the soles of the feet blistered after about five days! I followed her "cure" after that for at least five years and I then lost track of her. Cancer is one of the illnesses for which spiritual healing is one of the best approaches.

CANDIDIASIS/YEAST INFECTIONS (VAGINAL)
All Basics plus "Enhancing Immune Function" instructions.

There have been several published reports showing that a 600-mg. boric acid vaginal suppository provides symptomatic relief in just twenty-four hours. It usually takes about ten days of treatment (one 600-mg. suppository capsule inserted in the morning and another in the evening to wipe out the infection). If the problem returns, a repeated course of treatment of two to three days might be needed.

One study compared boric-acid suppositories to the common drug nystatin. Boric acid was far superior, with a 96 percent cure rate compared to a 64 percent cure rate with nystatin.[112]

Both the capsules and the boric acid are available at pharmacies.

CHOLESTEROL/CORONARY ARTERY DISEASE
There is no circumstance under which I would take any of the cholesterol-lowering drugs. They are dangerous, and it is another experiment like Prempro® that may not be revealed until thousands have suffered complications and/or death.

What to do?

• Relax ten to fifteen minutes twice daily.

- Exercise—build to an hour a day.
- Avoid like the plague all margarines and artificially hardened fats.
- Avoid "fast foods" and carbonated drinks.
- Go on a low-carbohydrate diet.
- Avoid homogenized milk. That makes the fat much more dangerous.
- Use *only* butter, olive oil, and flax-seed oil as added fats.
- Drink plenty of real water—not chlorinated/fluoridated.

Take:

- Beta sitosterol complex, 1,200 to 4,200 mg. daily

If not better in one month, add Lecithin granules, 2 heaping tablespoons twice daily.

If this has not worked in one month add one at a time:

Arginine, up to 6 grams daily
Taurine, up to 4,000 mg. at bedtime
Co-Q 10, 200 mg. daily

Eat lots of fruits and vegetables.

Check your homocysteine level; it is ten times as important as cholesterol and easily controlled with extra vitamin B_{12} and folic acid.

CHRONIC FATIGUE SYNDROME/FIBROMYALGIA
(*See also "Electromagnetic Dysthymia" below.*)

Use the complete "Anxiety/Panic Disorder" and "Depression" regimens, plus "DHEA Restoration."

COMPREHENSIVE MANAGEMENT FOR CHRONIC PAIN
AND DIFFICULT DISEASES—INCLUDING FAILED
BACK SURGERY, THALAMIC PAIN SYNDROME,
POST-HERPETIC NEURALGIA

Always use the SheLi TENS™ first, including the Ring of Earth. If that proves inadequate, then find a competent, charismatic, and compassionate holistic physician, who selects the team and employs:

NO mood-altering or pain-relieving drugs

Cranial electrical stimulation

TENS

Biofeedback, autogenic training, and related self-regulation techniques

Computerized traction with IDD®

Massage

Heat and cold

Hot tubs

Vibratory music beds

Acupuncture

Humanistic psychological approaches

Good nutrition, including supplements

Physical exercise, including yoga and free-form tai chi

DEPRESSION (INCLUDING BIPOLAR DISORDER)

Add to Basics plus "Anxiety" suggestions:

1. Meat broth (as described in chapter 4): 8 ounces of stew-sized meat, cooked overnight in a slow cooker, low heat,

with 1 quart water, 2 tablespoons vinegar, and seasonings to taste. Drink at least two cups daily.

2. Photostimulation: The Shealy RelaxMate™ one hour daily

3. Use the Liss TENS, Shealy Series™ transcranially for forty to sixty minutes daily or use the Liss or the SheLi TENS™ on the Ring of Fire. Prescriptions are required for either of these.

4. Listen to great classical music at least one hour daily.

5. If not doing well after a month, add lithium orotate, 45 mg. daily (bipolars should start with this).

6. Tryptophan, 1,000 mg. and up to at least 5,000 mg. per day, is actually wonderful for most depressed people.

7. Stimulation of the Ring of Fire with the SheLi TENS™ works better than any other *single* approach.

8. Holos® Wellness Centers offer these treatments.

DHEA RESTORATION

There are four excellent techniques for restoration of DHEA, highly recommended. Unless you have a serious disease such as Lupus, I do not recommend taking DHEA supplements. And do not ever take DHEA supplements if you have cancer of the prostate, breast, uterus, or ovaries.

The four techniques are all safe and work independently of one another, each adding to the others:

1. Ring of Fire stimulation with the SheLi TENS™. Obviously you could use acupuncture, but it is much less expensive in the long run to buy the stimulator and use it.

2. See my booklet *DHEA: The Youth and Health Hormone*

OR the book *The Methuselah Potential for Health and Longevity* (888-242-6105).

3. Natural Progesterone Cream, one-quarter teaspoon twice daily on the skin. I do not recommend this for patients with the cancers listed above.
4. Dr. sHEALy's Youth Formula®, 4 tablets daily
5. Biogenics® Magnesium Lotion, 4 to 6 teaspoons on skin daily

DIABETES
Add to Basics:

Adjust Body Mass Index between 18 and 24
Use low-glycemic-index foods
Gymnema sylvestra, 500 mg., two to three times daily
Tri-chromium complex, 1,000 micrograms, daily
Deep relaxation 30 minutes daily
Exercise: Build to one hour daily

ELECTROMAGNETIC DYSTHYMIA (EMD)
(Chronic Fatigue; Fibromyalgia)
EMD is a generalized disorder of chronic fatigue, anxiety, depression, and a significantly weakened immune system. It is rarely diagnosed and goes under the rubric of environmental allergies, candidiasis, chronic fatigue, M-E (in England), REDD syndrome, etc. All these problems are associated with deficiency in DHEA, magnesium, and essential amino acids, especially tryptophan and taurine.

Thus, use all the basic recommendations as well as those for "Anxiety/Panic Disorder," "Depression," and "Enhancing Immune Function," including especially use of the SheLi TENS™ activation of the Ring of Fire.

ENDOMETRIOSIS
Keep your Body Mass Index below 25!
Use Eugesterone cream from day 10 to day 28 of cycle, or
    start of next cycle.
Use stress-reduction techniques.

ENHANCING IMMUNE FUNCTION
All Basics plus:

All "DHEA Restoration" as above, plus daily:
Glucan, 2 tablespoons
Co-Q 10, 400 mg.
Maxogenol™, 4 tablets
Glutamine powder, one teaspoon with each meal
Thymuril (thymus extract), 4 tablets
Coconut oil, 3 tablespoons daily
Castor oil packs to the abdomen
Autogenic training (my Basic Schultz tape)
90 Days to Stress-Free Living book

FIBROMYALGIA—
SEE "ELECTROMAGNETIC DYSTHYMIA"

FIVE SACRED RINGS *(described in earlier chapters)*
Over the past ten years I have discovered in the human body five circuits that activate specific chemical pathways. The stimulation

required appears to be that of either the Liss TENS® or the SheLi TENS™. In general the SheLi TENS™ is more effective in some situations, which will be mentioned below, but either may work. For those individuals who are very sensitive to electrical current, the Liss may be more easily accepted. The Liss puts out 15,000 pulses per second, modulated 15 and 500 times per second. The SheLi puts out all frequencies, including 54 to 78 billion pulses per second. This latter frequency is that which has been proven by Ukrainian physicists to equal the frequency of human DNA. Regular TENS and the AlphaStim® did not raise DHEA.

The circuits are:

FIRE, which increases DHEA, the adrenal hormone that is low or deficient in most individuals because of excess stress. In addition to raising DHEA, stimulation of FIRE has been clinically successful in 70 to 80 percent of patients who have rheumatoid arthritis, migraine, depression, or diabetic neuropathy. Stimulation must be done daily for three months and then at least twice a week to maintain the improvement. The points are: K 3; CV 2, 6, and 18; B 22; MH 6; LI 18; and GV 20. The SheLi TENS™ is the only one that works in diabetic neuropathy.

WATER, which optimizes aldosterone, the hormone responsible for regulation of water and potassium. Theoretically it may help balance emotions. *Combined with FIRE*, stimulation of WATER has been found to help significantly in weight loss. The points are: SP 4; GV 8, 20; CV 14; B 10, 13; H 7; and TH 16.

AIR, which raises neurotensin, a neurochemical that helps fat metabolism but is also a neuroleptic. This effect appears to assist in establishing a meditative state or "simultaneity of thought." The points are: SP 1A; LIV 3; S 36; LI; G 20; GV 1, 16, 20.

EARTH, which raises calcitonin significantly. Calcitonin is a hormone produced in the thyroid and is the key regulator of calcium metabolism in bone. Calcitonin is a powerful tool for maintaining strong bones. Calcitonin is also forty to sixty times as strong as morphine in reducing pain. Stimulation of this ring may help addiction, ground the personality, and be an adjunct in rebuilding the body. The points are: K 1; B 60, 54; LI 16; ST 9; SI 17; and GV 20.

CRYSTAL, which reduces free radicals significantly, within three days of starting daily stimulation, especially with the SheLi TENS™. Free radicals are the destructive chemicals that cause aging and degeneration. Theoretically, reducing free radicals could be the single most important adjunct for enhancing health and longevity. The SheLi TENS™ is more effective than the Liss. The points are: SP 4; GB 11, 30.5; CV 8.5, 14.5, 23; and GV 4.5, 7.5, 14.5, 20.

GROWTH HORMONE ACTIVATION/ANTIAGING

1. I *do not recommend* growth hormone itself. The commercial product Rejuvamax® has been shown to raise GH safely, especially if used daily with the Liss TENS™ transcranially.
2. Royal Maca, up to one tablespoon daily, has some excellent evidence for overall rejuvenation, including sometimes controlling all menopausal symptoms.
3. Regular use of Biogenics® Magnesium Lotion.
4. For men, *tribulus terrestris* 500 mg., four to eight times daily, to help restore testosterone production.
5. Wear a Clarus Q-Pendant. It protects you from 50 milligauss of EMF (888-242-6105).

HEADACHE

See "Migraine." In general, once competent medical evaluation has ruled out any other problem, most headaches will respond to the approaches given for migraine.

HYPERTENSION

Add to Basics:

Double the amount of Biogenics® Magnesium Lotion.

Calcium citrate, 1,000 to 1,500 mg. daily

Learn to warm feet to 96 degrees mentally!

Read and Practice *90 Days to Stress-Free Living* (book).

Consider vitamin D3, 2,000 units daily.

Co-Q 10, 200 to 300 mg. daily

Omega-3 Fatty acids, 4,000 to 6,000 mg. daily

Timed Release Arginine, 1,000 mg. twice a day

Arjuna, 500 mg. two to four times a day

HYPERTHYROIDISM

Eat broccoli, kale, cauliflower, cabbage, etc., daily.

Lemon Balm as tea or tincture, four times daily

Bugleweed, as tea or tincture, four times daily

Autogenic training—Basic Schultz tape twice daily

Castor-oil packs to thyroid

Double the basic dose of Biogenics® Magnesium Lotion.

Avoid caffeine, aspartame, etc.

HYPOTHYROIDISM

Iodine, Iodoral®, one tablet daily

If temperature does not return to normal, add SheLi
TENS™ on Ring of Fire.

IMPOTENCE
Always start with beta sitosterol 1,200 to 1,800 mg. daily.
If there is no severe vascular disease or neuropathy, then
the following may be useful:
Tribulus terrestris, 500 mg., up to 8 capsules daily
"DHEA Restoration," described above
Epimedium sagittatum, 100 mg., up to 6 capsules daily
Timed Release Arginine, 1 gram twice a day
If this does not work, try VigEros™ formula, which adds:
Xanthoparmelia scabrosa and Cnidium monnier

INSOMNIA
All Basics plus:
Liss TENS™, Shealy series, transcranially an hour daily
Taurine 3,000 mg. at bedtime
If not effective, try either one of the following one at a
time at bedtime, not both together:
Kava kava 750 mg. (This should not be used more than a
week at a time.)
Tryptophan up to 10 grams plus lithium orotate, 45 mg.

IRRITABLE BOWEL/LEAKY GUT/CROHN'S DISEASE
Always Basics, plus avoid wheat, corn, citrus, eggs, dairy products, peanuts, chocolate, aspartame, junk food, and carbonated
soft drinks. These patients often proceed into Electromagnetic
Dysthymia.

Add glutamine powder, one tablespoon, twice daily.
Roberts Complex or Compound, 4 capsules daily

Acidophilus, 5 capsules daily

Boswellin, 250 mg., 4 capsules daily

If not much better in a month, add Hanna Kroeger's Worm-wood Combination, 4 capsules daily and add two daily, building up to 14 daily for one month.

MACULAR DEGENERATION

All the Basics, plus "Enhancing Immune Function" approaches, as this is clearly a disease of excess free radicals and inadequate antioxidants.

Most important: chelated zinc, 30 mg.; taurine, 3,000 mg.; Co-Q 10, 100 mg.

In addition, there is good evidence that electrical stimulation with the Liss TENS™, of the closed eyes, ten minutes daily, is of benefit if started early.

I'd also recommend stimulation at least of the Ring of Fire and Ring of Crystal.

MENOPAUSAL SYMPTOMS

Add to Basics:

Start with natural progesterone cream, Eugesterone, one-quarter teaspoon twice daily on the skin. If ovaries have been re-moved or symptoms are not controlled, get a prescription from a compounding pharmacy for daily dose in two one-quarter tea-spoons of cream: 60-mg. of natural progesterone and 2.5 mg. of biest (estriol and estradiol).

If you are on Prempro® and want to come off:

Start with the Eugesterone cream and after three weeks cut your Prempro® dose in half. In another three weeks reduce by half every other day. After another three weeks reduce by half every third day. In another three weeks, stop altogether. If you have hot flashes, add Herbal Balance-F, three daily. This product contains the effective herbal proestrogens.

If the herbal preparation does not work, then you need a prescription, to be filled at a compounding pharmacy, containing in a daily total dose of two one-quarter teaspoons 60 mg. of natural progesterone and 2.5 mg. of biest (estriol and estradiol). I do not recommend estrone. Rarely, testosterone may be needed also and may be added to the cream.

Do autogenic training—Basic Schultz tape.

MEUNIERE'S SYNDROME
Always Basics with plenty of magnesium. Try avoiding wheat, milk products, citrus, egg, corn, chocolate, peanuts. (Food allergies may be a major contributor.)

Cocculus (a homeopathic remedy) may help.

Acupuncture is one option.

Finally, stimulation of the Ring of Air with the SheLi TENS™ should be tried if all else fails.

METHUSELAH PROMISE:
HEALTHY YOUTHING
In addition to the Ring of Fire, stimulation of the Rings of Crystal and Earth should optimize overall health and longevity. The SheLi TENS™ is ideal for this. The Ring of Earth increases calcitonin—great for bone strength and general well-being. The Ring of Crystal markedly reduces free radicals, the cause of disease, aging, and death!

MIGRAINE
Add to Basics:

1. Temperature biofeedback. Those who *learn* to raise the temperature of the index finger to 96 degrees mentally within five minutes reduce the severity and frequency of migraine headaches by 84 percent.
2. Ring of Fire: Stimulation daily with the Liss TENS™ reduces frequency by 75 percent, almost twice as good as the "best" drug for prophylaxis, Depakote®, which has *many* complications. Indeed, I will not recommend that drug.
3. Computerized cervical traction: daily for two weeks. Excellent adjunct that reduces or eliminates many types of headache.
4. Autogenic training, even without biofeedback, is extremely useful.
5. Food sensitivities: Two-thirds of migraineurs reduce frequency markedly by avoiding wheat, corn, eggs, citrus, milk products, peanuts, chocolate, red wine, cheese, and pickled herring. After six weeks or so, if headaches are markedly improved, add back one of these food groups each week to see which must be permanently avoided.
6. *No* aspartame; no smoking; no carbonated soft drinks.
7. Biogenics® Magnesium Lotion. All migraineurs are deficient in magnesium.
8. Riboflavin, vitamin B$_2$, 400 mg. daily, is helpful in some patients.

9. Natural progesterone cream, one-quarter teaspoon on skin twice daily from tenth to twenty-eighth day of cycle or until next cycle begins, whichever is earliest.

10. Get and follow recommendations in my book *90 Days to Stress-Free Living*.

11. Tryptophan 1,000 mg., three or four times daily, plus 45 mg. of lithium orotate, is often helpful.

12. Taurine, 1,000 mg., three times daily, may be helpful.

MULTIPLE SCLEROSIS, AMYOTROPHIC LATERAL SCLEROSIS (ALS)

Use all the "Enhancing Immune Function" tools plus the SheLi TENS™ on Sacred Rings; I'd use Rings of Fire, Earth, and Crystal.

OBESITY

Always check your temperature before getting out of bed. If it is consistently below 97.6° F, you have relative hypothyroidism, and 1,500 mcg. of iodine daily for a month may help. If not, add the Ring of Fire.

In general, the Barnes diet works best for most people. It consists of a maximum of two servings of bread and one small serving of fruit total per day plus unlimited eggs, meat of all kinds, and nonstarchy vegetables.

For those who are recalcitrant to Barnes, the rice diet is recommended: unlimited rice and canned fruits! Repulsive after a while, but it works!

Increase your exercise slowly over several months to at least one hour daily.

Finally, the Rings of Fire and Water each day may help.

Attitude and activity are essential! And NO aspartame.

Obsessive-Compulsive Disorder
Before going on drugs, do the Basics, plus the "Anxiety" and the "Depression" regimens and:

Add lithium orotate, 45 mg. daily; and tryptophan, 1,000 mg., three to four times daily.

Osteoporosis
* SheLi TENS™ on Ring of Earth

Plus:

* Calcium citrate, 1,500 mg.
* Double the dose of Biogenics® Magnesium Lotion
* Boron, 3 mg.
* Vitamin D, 800 to 1,000 units
* Exercise

Prostate Problems
(Benign Prostatic Hypertrophy [BPH] or Cancer)
Always the Basics plus:

* Drink at least 2 quarts of good water daily.
* Take small flower willow tea, 3 cups daily, for at least two weeks yearly.
* Beta sitosterol, 3,000 to 4,200 mg. daily
* Pygeum, 50 mg., 2 to 10 daily
* Nettles capsules, 2 twice daily
* Cernilton, 4 to 8 tablets daily

With cancer, use "Enhancing Immune Function" (described above).

Stay sexually active! Use it or lose it! If you do not have a partner, masturbate and enjoy it.

In chronic prostatitis, but not cancer, prostate massage at least three times weekly.

PSORIASIS

All the usual health-enhancing approaches.

This autoimmune disease of the skin often responds very well to a diet of two meals daily of raw vegetables, fruits, seeds, and nuts. The third meal should be broiled or baked fish with steamed vegetables and brown rice. Use a tablespoon or two of raw flaxseed oil over the vegetables and/or rice.

Biogenics® Magnesium Lotion—apply on *normal* skin only.

ROSACEA

Basics plus:

"Enhancing Immune Function" (described above) plus:

Try eliminating wheat, corn, eggs, dairy, citrus, chocolate, and peanuts for one month. If you improve add one food at a time, one a week, to see if there is a specific causal agent.

Apply Emu oil to skin twice daily. If that does not work, try jojoba oil.

SEUTERMAN HOMEOPATHY

This approach uses six homeopathic agents during each treatment:

- Traditional homeopathic
- Nosode

- Krebs cycle
- Quinone
- Detox
- Organ tissue

If you are interested in my protocol for rheumatoid and auto-immune diseases, e-mail me with a request and your regular mailing address (normshealy@normshealy.net).

SHINGLES

If started early, either amantadine or ramantadine is worth trying, along with at least 6 grams of vitamin C and 100 mg. of vitamin B complex.

Once postherpetic shingles pain starts, the treatment of choice is the SheLi TENS™ with electrodes above and below the scar. If that does not work, try the Ring of Earth.

UTERINE FIBROIDS

In general this problem is the result of long years of estrogen dominance. It is best treated with natural progesterone cream, one-quarter teaspoon twice daily on the skin from the tenth to the twenty-eighth day of cycle or the start of the next cycle.

Also, keep your weight at 23 to 24 Body Mass Index. Fatty tissue contributes estrogen!

Exercise vigorously, building up to the equivalent of four miles of brisk walking in one hour at least five days a week.

Stimulation of the Ring of Fire with a Liss or SheLi TENS™ is also of potential benefit. You might consult a healer. This is the type of problem that may respond to spiritual healing.

• • •

I HAVE SPENT HALF A CENTURY EXPLORING HEALTH AND am convinced that you control both health and longevity. If you are willing to make the healthy choices discussed in this book, you have a remarkable opportunity to enjoy *Life Beyond 100*. The secret of the Fountain of Youth is now in your hands. True youthful aging is the future for those who care enough to follow a healthy life path. Join me in continuing a fun journey.

THE DAILY DOZEN EXERCISES

 ## 1. *Good-Morning Exercise*

A. Stand with feet shoulder-width apart.

B. Bend forward in a relaxed manner, exhaling and loosening the shoulders, neck, and hands.

C. Raise up and stretch while inhaling deeply, head up, back arched, on tiptoes. Repeat seven times.

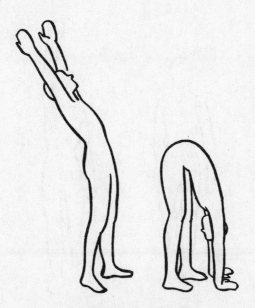

GOOD-MORNING EXERCISE

2. Jangle

A. Jog in place while loosening the shoulders, neck, hands, and lower extremities. Continue until breathing is well accelerated.

B. Alternately raise the arms overhead (still jogging) and stretch, making a clenched fist.

C. Inhale deeply, holding each clenched fist at the top for several running steps. Repeat five to ten times with each hand. (Concentrate on deep inhalation.)

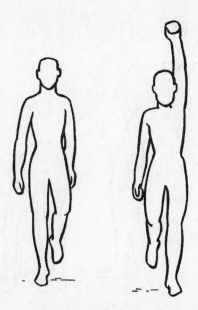

JANGLE

3. Shoulder Shrugs

A. Raise the arms forward and shoulders up, then arms overhead, continuing through in a complete circle. Do seven to twelve repetitions.

B. Reverse the motion and circle back seven to twelve times.

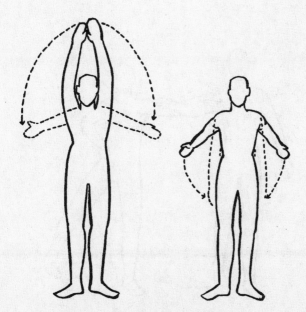

SHOULDER SHRUGS

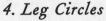

4. Leg Circles

A. Stand on left leg while holding on to a firm object for balance (not necessary if you have good balance).

B. Extend right leg forward with knee straight about twelve to sixteen inches.

C. Turn toes inward. Then, keeping the knee straight and foot in, move the leg an equal distance to the rear.

D. Circle the leg outward (laterally) about twenty-four to thirty-six inches, then forward again.

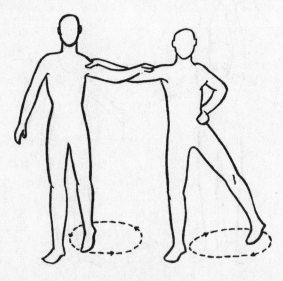

LEG CIRCLES

5. *Arm Circles*

A. Extend right arm forward.

B. Turn thumb toward the ground.

C. Raise arm overhead and swing through in a circle, keeping the elbow straight, for ten to twelve repetitions.

D. Reverse the motion and do ten to twelve repetitions. Repeat with the opposite arm.

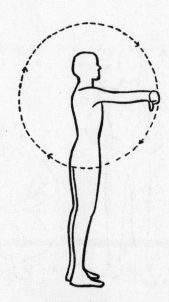

ARM CIRCLES

6. *Knee Bends on Toes*

A. Begin with hands on the hips. For someone who has difficulty at first, place the hands farther down the thighs for leverage. Stand with feet shoulder width apart, with head up, back straight.

B. Exhale as you squat down.

C. Inhale as you come up. Bounce slightly at the bottom before coming up. Concentrate on three counts—it's down on *one, two* with the bounce, and up on *three*. Repeat seven times.

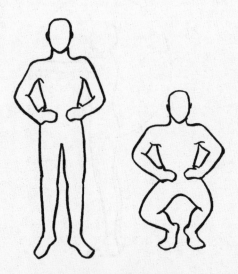

KNEE BENDS ON TOES

7. *The Barnyard Shuffle Loosener*

A. Stand on one foot. Bend forward at the waist.

B. Extend the opposite arm forward and the loose leg to the rear. Vigorously shake both hand and foot as if they had something on them that you wanted shaken off.

C. Reverse legs and repeat two to three times each.

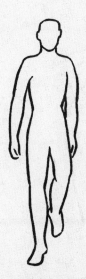

THE BARNYARD SHUFFLE LOOSENER

8. Hip Circle or Hula Hoop

A. For the hip circle the feet are placed parallel, a bit wider than shoulder width apart.

B. Bring the hips well forward, clasp hands behind the back, then circle the hips, keeping the head and shoulders relatively stationary, trying to make a perfect circle. (It's as if you were standing in a barrel and trying to touch all sides as you go around.) This is to develop flexibility in the pelvic girdle and loosen up the lower back. Repeat seven times in each direction.

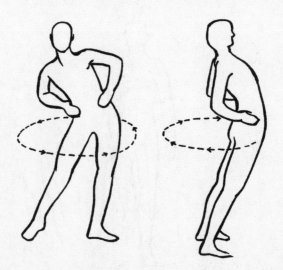

HIP CIRCLE OR HULA HOOP

9. Forward Bends (Knees Bent)

A. Place the feet wider than shoulder width apart with the toes pointed inward.

B. Bend forward at the waist, exhaling, bending as far as you can comfortably on *one,* then stretch farther forward on *two, three,* and *four.*

C. Raise up and stretch backward with the hands on the hips, then return. Repeat seven times.

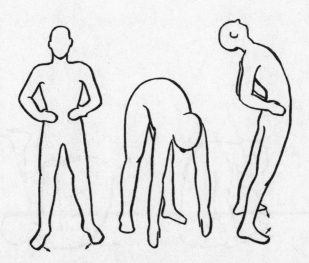

FORWARD BENDS (KNEES BENT)

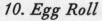

10. Egg Roll

A. In a seated position grasp the hands behind the knees, crossing the feet if desired.

B. Keeping the chin down on the chest, raise the knees, and roll back on the shoulders while exhaling.

C. Roll back and forth, up and down, on the spine, returning forward to the seated position each time. Repeat seven times.

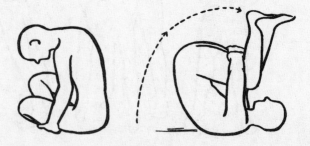

EGG ROLL

11. Cervical Release (for lymphatic drainage)

A. While sitting, place thumb and forefinger together in back of the neck, at the base of the skull.

B. Raise the chin, then press the fingertips firmly in the hollow-most spot, or so-called "nape" of the neck, near the midline. This will be the area of the third cervical. The fourth and fifth vertebrae, just below, stick out prominently. Keep the pressure above them.

C. Lie back in a relaxed manner with knees up, chin raised, and continue the pressure two to four minutes, massaging any sore spots you may find there.

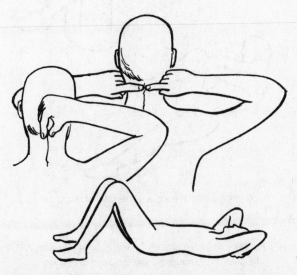

CERVICAL RELEASE (FOR LYMPHATIC DRAINAGE)

12. *Alternate Knee and Elbow Touch*

A. While still lying down, clasp hands behind the neck.

B. Raise the knees.

C. Alternatively twist the torso, touching the elbows to the *inside* of the opposite knee. (The leg not being touched should extend straight out, toes pointed, slightly above the ground.) Repeat ten to twelve times.

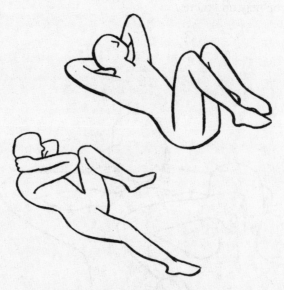

ALTERNATE KNEE AND ELBOW TOUCH

Daily Dozen: from *The Over-29 Health Book,* by Jeffrey Furst (Donning Publishers, Norfolk, VA, 1979). Reprinted with permission from Dr. Genevieve Haller.

GLOSSARY

acetylcholine: A neurotransmitter that is the primary facilitator of activity in the parasympathetic or vegetative nervous system.

acupuncture meridian: There are twelve major acupuncture meridians, which are the energetic circuits connecting acupuncture points.

adrenals: Small glands located on the top of each kidney and responsible for manufacturing "adrenaline" or epinephrine, norepinephrine, dopamine, cortisol, aldosterone, and some small amounts of testosterone, etc.

aerobic points: A system of measuring the oxygen consumption of various physical activities to give an indication of health benefits.

aldosterone: An adrenal-produced hormone that helps regulate water and potassium metabolism.

alpha range: Electrical frequency of the brain that is in a state of relaxation, eight to twelve cycles per second.

andropause: The male equivalent of menopause. Around age fifty men begin to produce less testosterone.

angina pectoris: Pain in the chest associated with coronary artery insufficiency or disease.

autogenic training: A systematic form of self-hypnosis devised by J. H. Schultz and very useful for obtaining self-control over many stress illnesses.

beta-blockers: Drugs that block one of the primary adrenal stress hormones.

beta stage: The electrical frequency of the brain when one is alert, generally in a range of thirteen to twenty-six cycles per second.

bioelectromagnetism: The flow of electricity produces a magnetic field. Bioelectromagnetism is the electromagnetic pattern produced by life, particularly in human beings.

biofeedback: The feedback to an individual of any electrical, chemical, or physiological change taking place in the body. The feedback can be in the form of audio or visual signals that allow one to gain control over that physiological response.

calcitonin: A hormone produced by the thyroid gland; it is essential for maintaining the strength of the skeleton.

chakras: Specific energy centers associated with various parts of the body. There are seven major chakras, the lower six of which are correlated with concentrations of nerve energy such as the sciatic plexus, pelvic plexus, solar plexus, heart plexus, cervical and neck plexus, and brain. The seventh chakra is the connection with the soul or spirit.

chi (qi): The theoretical, universal life force, which flows in the acupuncture meridians.

chloride waters: Natural spring waters that contain significant amounts of chlorine.

chloro-carbonate waters: Natural spring waters, which naturally contain chlorine and carbon dioxide.

chronic fatigue: The clinical status in which the individual has a marked reduction in energy. It is associated with a wide variety of other symptoms, primarily including depression.

circadian rhythm: The natural biological variations in hormones and the physiology of the body.

cnidium monnier: A Chinese herb that is thought to assist in penile erections.

cortisol: The major hormone produced by the adrenal glands and responsible for assisting in maintaining a healthy immune system.

cytokinase: An enzyme that breaks down cytokines, hormone-like proteins secreted by many cells; cytokines regulate the intensity and duration of immune response and are involved in cell-to-cell communication.

delta: The slowest of brain electrical activities from one to three cycles per second, associated with very deep states of relaxation and detachment.

DHEA: Dehydroepiandrosterone, the single most important hormone for measuring or evaluating total stress reserves.

diastolic: The "lower" blood pressure, which represents the state at which the heart is filling with blood or relatively resting after a contraction.

electroencephalogram (EEG): The electrical activity of the brain.

electromagnetic dysthymia (EMD): A clinical state associated with depression and generalized problems of symptoms including chronic fatigue, many immune dysfunctions, etc.

electromagnetic frequencies (EMF): The frequencies involved in the broad spectrum of light and sound.

electromagnetism: The magnetic field produced by the flow of electrical current.

estrogen: Hormones primarily produced in the ovary including estrone, estradiol, and estriol.

etheric body: An energetic field around the human body believed to be related to the electromagnetic reflections of the body.

ferro-manganese waters: Natural spring waters that contain iron and manganese.

5-alpha reductase: An enzyme that converts testosterone to dihydrotestosterone.

5-hydroxyindoleacetic acid (5-HIAA): The breakdown product of serotonin.

Five Sacred Rings: Five separate electrical circuits in the body involving acupuncture points. These include specific rings that, when stimulated appropriately, increase DHEA, aldosterone, neurotensin, and calcitonin or selectively decrease free radicals.

free radicals: Chemical products in the body that are physiologically and electrically active. They tend to "oxidize" or break down tissue. Many of them are products of fat metabolism.

gamma hydroxybutyrate: A chemical that induces a deep state of sleep.

giga-energy: Frequencies at billions of cycles per second.

Giga-Tens™: An electrical stimulator that generates frequencies at fifty-four to seventy-eight billion cycles per second, the frequency of human DNA.

gold iodide crystals: Dull black or brown crystals of gold combined with iodide.

gonadal dysfunction: The gonads are the organs that produce sex cells; testes in men or the ovary in women. Dysfunction means that they are not producing hormones, sperm, or eggs appropriately.

GSR (galvanic skin response): This is essentially the electrical resistance of the skin.

histidine: A basic amino acid found in most proteins.

holism: A broad concept that the whole is greater than the sum of the parts.

homocysteine: An abnormal protein that represents an incomplete breakdown of the essential amino acid methionine. It is extremely harmful and increases the risk of arteriosclerosis and hardening of the arteries, as well as damage to the brain and nervous system.

HRT (hormone replacement therapy): The use of various estrogens, progesterones, or testosterones to replace the hormones lost after menopause or andropause.

human DNA restoration: DNA is the basic chromosomal material that is associated with genes. Genes are damaged by various influences including free radicals. Human DNA restoration is a technique for rejuvenating and restoring DNA to its normal healthy status.

hyperinsulinemia: An excess production of insulin.

iatrogenic complications: Complications of treatments by physicians.

IGF-1 (insulin-like growth hormone factor-1): Chemicals other than insulin that are associated with immune function.

IL-6/interleukin-6: A lymphokine derived from fibroblasts, microphages, and tumor cells that increases production and secretion of immuneglobulin, enhancing immune strength.

immune dysregulation: Malfunction of a normal immune system.

isoleucine: One of the essential amino acids.

L-arginine: One of the critical amino acids that helps produce nitrous oxide, a chemical regulating blood flow and also one of the foundation molecules for making growth hormone.

L-cells: Concepts of particular cells associated with life.

L-field: The electromagnetic field produced by living tissue.

leucine: An essential amino acid.

limbering: Stretching to increase flexibility.

Liss stimulator: A particular electrical stimulator that puts out frequencies of 15,000 cycles modulated five hundred and fifteen times per second. Used particularly for treating depression.

Liss TENS™, Shealy Series: A particular model of the Liss stimulator used by Dr. Shealy to treat depression.

lysine: An essential amino acid.

magnesium taurate: A combination of magnesium with the amino acid taurine.

malondialdehyde (MDA): A chemical used to measure the concentration of free radicals in the urine.

melatonin: Melatonin is a hormone important in regulation of sleep and also associated with immune function.

methionine: One of the essential amino acids.

Minnesota Multiphasic Personality Inventory (MMPI): The most widely used written test to evaluate the personality.

natural progesterone cream: A cream applied to the skin that contains the natural hormone progesterone, a hormone produced in both men and women and one of the major precursors of cortisol, testosterone, and estrogen.

negative polarity: Electrical current may produce either positive or negative waves. Negative polarity is the negative phase of electrical current.

neurotensin: A natural neurochemical produced in the brain and other parts of the nervous system. It is a normal chemical that helps induce a deep state of relaxation and detachment from worry.

norepinephrine: The major stress hormone, part of the adrenaline complex, which raises blood pressure and pulse.

orgone: Dr. Wilhelm Reich's concept of life energy.

ornithine: An important amino acid.

parasympathetic nervous system: The vegetative nervous system that is associated with rest, digestion, and recuperation.

phenylalanine: An essential amino acid.

photostimulation: Lights flashed onto the skin or into the eyes at specific frequencies.

positive polarity: The positive phase of an electrical current.

pregnenolone: Sometimes called the "mother hormone" as it is the first major hormone in the sequences that proceed from cholesterol through pregnenolone to produce progesterone, DHEA, cortisol, estrogen, testosterone, and progesterone.

progesterone: A hormone produced in both men and women that is one of the precursors of cortisol, testosterone, and estrogen.

prostate disease: The prostate is a gland in the male that produces most of the fluid in male ejaculate. Many diseases may affect the prostate including infections, abnormal growth, and cancer.

quartz crystal: A natural crystal occurring in many parts of the world; a major feature of quartz is piezoelectric, which means that a physical pressure on the quartz produces an electrical current.

radioactive appliance: This particular device described originally by Edgar Cayce actually does not produce radioactivity. It is sometimes called the radial device and is basically used to balance electrical current throughout the body.

REM: Rapid eye movements produced during dreaming.

Ring of Air: An electrical circuit in the body involving thirteen specific acupuncture points that, when appropriately stimulated, produce neurotensin.

Ring of Crystal: An electrical circuit in the body involving thirteen specific acupuncture points that, when appropriately stimulated, decrease free radicals.

Ring of Earth: An electrical circuit in the body involving thirteen specific acupuncture points that, when appropriately stimulated, increase calcitonin.

Ring of Fire: An electrical circuit in the body involving twelve specific acupuncture points that, when appropriately stimulated, raise dehydroepiandrosterone or DHEA.

Ring of Water: An electrical circuit in the body involving thirteen specific acupuncture points that, when appropriately stimulated, increase aldosterone.

Sacred Rings of Life: The five specific electrical circuits associated with the most important neurochemical processes.

serotonin: A neurochemical produced in the brain and other parts of the body. It is particularly associated with mental alertness and mood.

Shealy RelaxMate II™: A pair of battery-operated glasses that produce flashes of light between one and seven cycles per second.

Sulphato-carbonate waters: Natural spring waters containing sulfur and carbon dioxide.

suprachiasmatic nucleus (SCN): A collection of brain cells above the projections of the optic nerve, the nerves of vision.

sympathetic nervous system: The fight-or-flight part of the nervous system that responds to stress.

Syndrome X: A combination of symptoms in individuals who are beginning to have problems metabolizing sugar properly. It is associated with obesity and a prediabetic condition.

systolic: The pressure of blood during the contraction of the heart.

taurine: An essential amino acid that plays an important role in regulating electrical potential in cells and helps stabilize the nervous system.

temperature control: The body normally maintains very narrow ranges of healthy temperature ranging from approximately 97.6 F during deep sleep to 98.6 F during normal daytime activity.

testosterone: The major male hormone.

theta waves: Electrical frequencies of the brain associated with creative visualization at four to seven cycles per second.

threonine: An amino acid associated with enhanced immune function.

trace elements: Extremely small amounts of materials required for healthy metabolism.

transdermal magnesium: Magnesium chloride applied to the skin.

tribulus terrestris: An herb that assists in production of testosterone.

tryptophan: An essential amino acid that is the precursor for production of serotonin.

tyrosine: An essential amino acid important in the production of adrenaline and the thyroid hormones.

valine: An essential amino acid.

VigEros™: An herbal combination for enhancement of male libido.

Wet Cell Battery: A device recommended by Edgar Cayce for helping to balance the nervous system.

xanthoparmelia scabrosa: An herb that assists in producing nitrous oxide to enhance penile erection.

Zung Self-Assessment Scale for Depression: One of the standard written psychological tests to determine whether or not one is depressed.

APPENDIX C

ZUNG SELF-ASSESSMENT SCALE FOR DEPRESSION

Name _____ Sex _____ Date _____

Age _____

	None OR a Little of the Time	Some of the Time	Good Part of the Time	Most OR All of the Time
1. I feel downhearted, blue, and sad	1	2	3	4
2. Morning is when I feel the best	4	3	2	1
3. I have crying spells or feel like it	1	2	3	4
4. I have trouble sleeping through the night	1	2	3	4
5. I eat as much as I used to	4	3	2	1
6. I enjoy looking at, talking to, and being with attractive women/men	4	3	2	1
7. I notice that I am losing weight	1	2	3	4
8. I have trouble with constipation	1	2	3	4
9. My heart beats faster than usual	1	2	3	4
10. I get tired for no reason	1	2	3	4
11. My mind is as clear as it used to be	4	3	2	1
12. I find it easy to do the things I used to do	4	3	2	1
13. I am restless and can't keep still	1	2	3	4
14. I feel hopeful about the future	4	3	2	1
15. I am more irritable than usual	1	2	3	4
16. I find it easy to make decisions	4	3	2	1
17. I feel that I am useful and needed	4	3	2	1
18. My life is pretty full	4	3	2	1
19. I feel that others would be better off if I were dead	1	2	3	4
20. I still enjoy the things I used to do	4	3	2	1

SDS Raw Score

On the facing page is a Zung test for depression. Complete the test, honestly assessing how you feel *right now*.

Now look at your total score. If it is 32 to 39, you have a sub-clinical depressive tendency. At least 40 percent of Americans fall into this range on the Zung. *Now* is the time to treat yourself vigorously, to prevent clinical depression. Take Azenda® for one month. If it changes your mood and feeling, nothing else is needed. Stay on Azenda. It is the best-quality SAM-E, a safe, natural product I recommend.

If your score is 40 or above (another 40 percent of Americans), you may try Azenda. If your score does not decrease significantly in a month, you need non-drug safe treatment with the SheLi TENS™ and RelaxMate, in addition to the supplements listed in chapter 7. You may have your physician contact me for more information, at normshealy@normshealy.net.

ACKNOWLEDGMENTS

If I listed all who have assisted me in this book, the list would be longer than the book! Perhaps it all started when I chose my parents. I have often said I did not have the courage to choose abusive parents. Both my parents nurtured me and gave me the blessings and support to explore life. My mother in her ninety-fourth year is still active and clear as a twenty-year-old. Her grandmother allowed me to read, at age twelve, the diary of my great-great-grandfather. I knew then that my life script called for over 100 years. Grandmother Rickard lived over 102 years. So, on my mother's side longevity is definitely part of genes and attitude. My father and four of his six brothers all died between forty-eight and fifty-four. They all smoked and had a few less-than-healthy habits. The sixth brother, a type-B laid-back person who worked outside, did not smoke, and had a wonderful attitude, lived to age eighty.

Beyond my own genetic family, the smartest choice of my life was my discovery forty-seven years ago of my wife of forty-six years, Mary-Charlotte, known as Chardy. Her support and love have sustained and encouraged me more than any other factor in this life. The additional blessings of three great children and five grandchildren have also increased the joy of life.

Innumerable teachers contributed to my passion for learning and research. Dr. Eugene Stead, Jr., Dr. Carl Moyer, Dr. Talmage Peele, and Sir John Eccles are among the scores of role models who helped refine my inquisitive nature. Numerous friends and scores of colleagues, almost as numerous as the patients I have seen, have widened my horizons even further. Dr. Genevieve Haller, Henry Rucker, Olga Worrall, Dr. Robert Leichtman, Dr. Saul Liss, and Caroline Myss have been at the forefront in my evolving consciousness. And, of course, the founding and continuing members of the American Holistic Medical Association have played a great role in my concepts and research. Edgar Cayce's Association for Research and Enlightment helped open my eyes in 1972 and has continued to stimulate my work. And Unity Church provided the positive foundation for my spiritual search. Buck Charlson, himself a creative genius, stimulated my search for understanding the mind and consciousness for almost three decades and supported my major research for a dozen years.

Finally, and certainly not least, the over thirty-five thousand patients of my career have provided me the challenges to pursue safe, effective alternatives to drugs and surgery. Most of my patients failed drugs and surgery before coming to me. Without their contributions, I could not know so much about so many variables of the human condition. Thank you!

In preparing this book through many incarnations, Jody Trotter, executive secretary supreme, has patiently retyped more times than any book yet. Lisa Munsat edited and polished well before I got the manuscript to the publisher. David Alexander wisely solicited Tarcher as the publisher. Mitch Horowitz, executive editor, went beyond the pale in assisting me to the final stage. And associate editor Ashley Shelby has been a wonderfully benign and careful final editor. May you all be with me to celebrate my 140th birthday! Thank all of you.

C. Norman Shealy, M.D., Ph.D.
Fair Grove, Missouri
June 20, 2005

NOTES

1. J. VanAuken, *Edgar Cayce's Approach to Rejuvenation of the Body* (Virginia Beach, VA: A.R.E. Press, 1996), 6.

2. Ibid., 7.

3. Ibid., 6,10,12,14.

4. Ibid., 23.

5. Ibid., 56.

6. Ibid., 73.

7. Eugene D. Robin, *Matters of Life and Death: Benefits of Medical Care* (New York: W. H. Freeman, 1984).

8. 2002 National Cancer Institute study, published in *Journal of the American Medical Association*, July 17, 2002.

9. J. E. Rossouw, G. L. Anderson, R. L. Prentice, et al. (writing group for Women's Health Initiative investigators), "Risks and Benefits of Estrogen plus Progestin in Healthy Postmenopausal Women: Principal Results from the Women's Health Initiative Randomized Controlled Trial," *JAMA*, July 17, 2002; 288: 321–333.

10. Robin, op. cit.

11. Tommy Thompson, speech delivered to the American Medical Association, July 18, 2002, Chicago.

12. "Investigators Find Repeated Deception in Ads for Drugs," *New York Times*, December 4, 2002.

13. S. N. Weingart et al., "Epidemiology of Medical Error," *British Med. J.* 310 (2000):774–77.

14. *Physicians' Desk Reference* (Montvale, N.J.: Medical Economics Co., 2001).

15. Robin, op. cit.

16. J. Gleick, *Faster: The Acceleration of Just About Everything* (New York: Pantheon, 1999).

17. Ibid.

18. Ibid.

19. H. Selye, *The Physiology and Pathology of Exposure to Stress* (Montreal: ACTA, Inc., 1950).

20. L. Orr, *Breaking the Death Habit: The Science of Everlasting Life* (Berkeley, Calif.: Frog Ltd., 1998).

21. Roy Walford, *Maximum Life Span* (New York: Norton, 1983).

22. G. Roth, M. Lane, D. Ingram, and S. Ball, "Studies Suggest Caloric Restriction in Monkeys May Extend Life," *J. Clin. Endocrin. and Metabolism* 82, no. 7 (1997):2093–96.

23. J. A. Mattson, M. A. Lane, G. S. Roth, and D. K. Ingram, *Exp. Gerontol.*, 2003, 38: 35–46.

24. C. N. Shealy and C. Norman, *DHEA: The Youth and Health Hormone* (Los Angeles: Keats Publishing, 1999), 44.

25. C. N. Shealy and C. M. Myss, *The Science of Medical Intuition* (Boulder, Colo.: Sounds True, 2002).

26. C. N. Shealy, *The Methuselah Potential for Health and Longevity* (Fair Grove, Mo.: Brindabella Books, 2002).

27. D. E. Antell and E. M. Taczanowski, "How Environment and Lifestyle Choices Influence the Aging Process," *Ann. Plast. Surg.* 43, no. 6 (Dec. 1999):585–88.

28. J. B. Carter, E. W. Banister, and A. P. Blaber, "Effect of Endurance Exercise on Autonomic Control of Heart Rate," *Sports Medicine* 33, no. 1 (2003):33–46.

29. J. Stevens, J. Cai, K. R. Evenson, and R. Thomas, "Fitness and Fatness as Predictors of Mortality from All Causes and from Cardiovascular Disease in Men and Women in the Lipid Research Clinics Study," *Am. Journal of Epidemiology* 156, no. 9 (Nov. 1, 2002):832–41.

30. E. Kahana, R. H. Lawrence, B. Kahana, K. Kercher, A. Wisniewski, E. Stoller, J. Tobin, and K. Stange, "Long-Term Impact of Preventive Proactivity on Quality of Life of the Old-Old," *Psychosom. Med.* 64, no. 3 (May–June 2002):382–94.

31. A. Drewnowski and W. J. Evana, "Nutrition, Physical Activity, and Quality of Life in Older Adults." Summary, *J. Gerontol. A. Biol. Sci. Med. Sci.* 56, Spec. no. 2 (October 2001):89–94.

32. R. S. Paffenbarger, Jr., S. N. Blair, and I. M. Lee, "A History of Physical Activity, Cardiovascular Health, and Longevity: The Scientific Contributions of Jeremy N. Morris, DSC, DPH, FRCP," *Int. J. Epidemiol.* 30, no. 5 (October 2001):1184–92.

33. S. N. Blair, Y. Cheng, and J. S. Holder, "Is Physical Activity or Physical Fitness More Important in Defining Health Benefits?" *Med. Sci. Sports Exerc.* 33, no. 6 Suppl. (June 2001): S379–99.

34. M. D. Ries, E. F. Philbin, and G. D. Groff, "Relationship Between Severity of Gonarthrosis and Cardiovascular Fitness," *Clin. Orthop.* 313 (April 1995):169–76.

35. I. M. Lee, C. C. Hsieh, and R. S. Paffenbarger, Jr., "Exercise Intensity and Longevity in Men: The Harvard Alumni Health Study," *JAMA* 273, no. 15 (Apr. 19, 1995):1179–84.

36. I. M. Lee and R. S. Paffenbarger, Jr., "Associations of Light, Moderate, and Vigorous Intensity Physical Activity with Longevity: The Harvard Alumni Study," *Am. J. Epidemiol.* 151, no. 3 (Feb. 1, 2000):293–99.

37. D. S. Khalsa, "Integrated Medicine and the Prevention and Reversal of Memory Loss," *Altern. Ther. Health Med.* 4, no. 6 (Nov. 1998):38–43.

38. E. R Eichner, "The Hematology of Inactivity," *Rheum. Dis. Clin. North Am.* 16, no. 4 (Nov. 1990):815–25.

39. L. Chernen, S. Friedman, N. Goldberg, A. Feit, T. Kwan, and R. Stein, "Cardiac Disease and Nonorganic Chest Pain: Factors Leading to Disability," *Cardiology* 86, no. 1 (1995):15–21.

40. H. Kraus, W. Nagler, and S. Weber, "Role of Exercise in the Prevention of Disease," *GP* 20, no. 3 (1959):121–26.

41. R. E. Anderson, T. A. Wadden, S. J. Bartlett, B. Zemel, T. J. Verde, and S. C. Franckowiak, "Effects of Lifestyle Activity vs. Structured Aerobic Exercise in Obese Women: A Randomized Trial," *JAMA* 281, no. 4 (1999):335–40.

42. A. L. Dunn, B. H. Marcus, J. B. Kampert, M. E. Garcia, H. W. Kohl, and S. N. Blair, "Comparison of Lifestyle and Structured Interventions to Increase Physical Activity and Cardiorespiratory Fitness: A Randomized Trial," *JAMA* 281, no. 4 (1999):327–34.

43. D. S. Butt, "The Sexual Response as Exercise," *Sports Med.* 9, no. 6 (1990):330–43.

44. A. J. Vita, R. B. Perry, H. B. Hubert, and J. F. Fries, "Aging, Health Risks, and Cumulative Disability," *N. Engl. J. Med.* 338, no. 15 (Apr. 9, 1998):1035–41.

45. Kenneth Cooper, *Aerobics* (New York: Bantam, 1973); *The Aerobics Way* (New York: Bantam, 1981); *The New Aerobics* (New York: Bantam, 1977).

46. Walter Kempner, "Compensation of Renal Metabolic Dysfunction: Treatment of Kidney Disease and Hypertensive Vascular Disease with the Rice Diet, III," *North Carolina Med. J.* 6 (1945):131–41.

47. R. C. Atkins, *Dr. Atkins' New Diet Revolution* (New York: HarperCollins, 2002).

48. G. Watson, *Nutrition and Your Mind: The Psychological Response* (New York: Bantam, 1978).

49. J. Chen, J. He, L. Hamm, V. Batuman, and P.K. Whelton, "Serum Antioxidant Vitamins and Blood Pressure in the United States Population," *Hypertension* 40 (2002):810.

50. T. Kozielcec, B. Starobrat-Hermelin, and L. Kotkowiak, "Deficiency of Certain Trace Elements in Children Lead to Hyperactivity," *Psychiatry Pol.* 28, no. 3 (1994):345–53; K. Suzuki, R. Oyama, E. Hayashi, and Y. Arakawa, "Liver Diseases and Essential Trace Elements," *Nippon Rinsho* 54, no. 1 (1996):85–92; A. N. Garg, V. Singh, R. G. Weginwar, and V. N. Sagdeo, "An Elemental Correlation Study in Cancerous and Normal Breast Tissue with Successive Clinical Stages by Neutron Activation Analysis," *Biol. Trace Elem. Res.* 46, no. 3 (1994):185–202.

51. M. Krachler, M. Lindschinger, B. Eber, N. Watzinger, and S. Wallner, "Trace Elements in Coronary Heart Disease: Impact of Intensified Lifestyle and Modification from Biological Trace Elements," *Biol. Trace Elem. Res.* 60 (1997):175–85.

52. B. T. Zhu, "Hyperhomocysteinemia Is a Risk Factor for Estrogen-Induced Hormonal Cancer," *Int. J. of Oncology* 22 (2003):499–508.

53. U. Lim and P. A. Cassano, "Homocysteine and blood pressure in the Third National Health and Nutrition Examination Survey, 1988–1994," *Am. J. Epidemiol.* 156, no. 12 (2002):1105–13.

54. B. Wang, L. Ma, and T. Liu, "406 Cases of Angina Pectoris in Coronary

Heart Disease Treated with Saponin of Tribulus Terrestris," *Zhong Xi Yi Jie He Za Zhi* 10, no. 2 (1990):85–87.

55. M. M. Merrill, J. C. Miller, J. J. Lipsitz, J. K. Walsh, and C. D. Wylie, "The Sleep of Long-Haul Truck Drivers," *NEJM* 337, no. 11 (1997):755–61.

56. Moore-Ede, *The Twenty-four Hour Society* (New York: Addison-Wesley, 1993).

57. Ibid.

58. "Men's Flab Linked to Lack of Deep Sleep," *Springfield News Leader*, August 16, 2000, Sec. B.

59. M. S. LaVert, M. Moore-Ede, and S. Campbell, *The Complete Idiot's Guide to Getting a Good Night's Sleep* (New York: Alpha Books, 1998).

60. J. Palmblad, B. Petrini, J. Wassereman, and T. Akerstedt, "Lymphocyte and Granulocyte Reactions During Sleep Deprivation," *Psychosomatic Med.* 41, no. 4 (1979):273–80.

61. J. Horne and A. J. Reid, "Night-time Sleep EEG Changes Following Body Heating in a Warm Bath," *Electroencephalography and Clin. Neurophysiology* 60 (1985):154–57.

62. M. Gillberg, "Sleepiness and Its Relation to the Length, Content, and Continuity of Sleep," *J. Sleep Res.* 4, no. 2 (1995):37–40.

63. A. J. Cleare, "The Neuroendocrinology of Chronic Fatigue Syndrome," *Endocr. Rev.* 24, no. 2 (2003):236–52.

64. C. Cajochen, K. Krauchi, and A. Wirz-Justice, "Role of Melatonin in the Regulation of Human Circadian Rhythms and Sleep," *J. Neuroendocrinol.* 15, no. 4 (2003):432–37.

65. D. P. Cardinali, M. G. Ladizesky, V. Boggio, R. A. Cutrera, and C. Mautalen, "Melatonin Effects on Bone: Experimental Facts and Clinical Perspectives," *J. Pineal Res.* 34, no. 2 (2003):81–87.

66. D. Aeschbach, L. Sher, T. T. Postolache, J. R. Matthews, M. A. Jackson, and T. A. Wehr, "A Longer Biological Night in Long Sleepers than in Short Sleepers," *J. Clin. Endocrinol. Metab.* 88, no. 1 (2003):26–30.

67. I. Arnulf, P. Quintin, J. C. Alvarez, L. Vigil, Y. Touitou, A. L Lebre, A. Bellenger, O. Varoquaux, J. P. Derenne, J. F. Allilaire, C. Benkelfat, and M. Leboyer, "Mid-morning Tryptophan Depletion Delays REM Sleep Onset in Healthy Subjects," *Neuropsychopharmacology* 27, no. 5 (2002):843–51.

68. K. Krauchi, C. Cajochen, E. Werth, and A. Wirz-Justice, "Alteration of In-

ternal Circadian Phase Relationships after Morning versus Evening Carbo-hydrate-Rich Meals in Humans," *J. Biol. Rhythms* 17, no. 4 (2002):364–76.

69. R. Luboshitzky, U. Ophir, R. Nave, R. Epstein, Z. Shen-Orr, and P. Herer, "The Effect of Pyridoxine Administration on Melatonin Secretion in Nor-mal Men," *Neuroendocrinol. Lett.* 23, no. 3 (2002):213–17.

70. N. Zisapel, "Melatonin-Dopamine Interactions: From Basic Neurochemistry to a Clinical Setting," *Cell Mol. Neurobiol.* 21, no. 6 (2001):605–16.

71. H. J. Eysenck, "Personality, Stress and Cancer," *British Journal of Medical Psychology* 61 (1988):57–75.

72. C. E. Ross and J. Moriwsky, "Family Relationships, Social Support, and Sub-jective Life Expectancy," *J. Health Soc. Behav.* 43, no. 4 (2002):469–89.

73. C. B. Thomas, K. R. Duszynski, and J. W. Shafer, "Family Attitudes Re-ported in Youth as Potential Predictors of Cancer," *Psychosomatic Med.* 41, no. 4 (1979):287–302.

74. J. K. Kiecolt-Glaser, L. McGuire, T. F. Robles, and R. Glaser, "Psychoneu-roimmunology: Psychological Influences on Immune Function and Health," *J. Consult. Clin. Psychol.* 70, no. 3 (2002):537–47.

75. J. K. Kiecolt-Glaser, L. McGuire, T. F. Robles, and R. Glaser, "Emotions, Morbidity, and Mortality: New Perspectives from Psychoneuroimmunol-ogy," *Annual Rev. Psychol.* 53 (2002):83–107.

76. A. R. Cappola, Q. L. Xue, L. Ferfucci, J. M. Guralnik, S. Volpato, and L. P. Fried, "Insulin-like Growth Factor I and Interleukin-6 Contribute Synergis-tically to Disability and Mortality in Older Women," *J. Clin. Endocrinol. Metab.* 88, no. 5(2003):2019–25.

77. M. G. Dik, S. M. Pluijm, C. Jonker, D. J. Deeg, M. Z. Lomecky, and P. Lips, "Insulin-like Growth Factor (IGF-1) and Cognitive Decline in Older Per-sons," *Neurobiol. Aging* 24, no. 2 (2003):573–81.

78. A. Figueroa, S. B. Going, L. A. Milliken, R. Blew, S. Sharp, and T. G. Lohman, "Body Composition Modulates the Effects of Hormone Replace-ment Therapy on Growth Hormone and Insulin-like Growth Factor-I Levels in Postmenopausal Women," *Gynecol. Obstet. Invest.* 54, no. 4 (2002):201–206.

79. D. K. Nias, "Therapeutic Effects of Low-Level Direct Electrical Currents," *Psychol. Bull.* 83 (1976):766.

80. N. Ishiko and W. R. Lowenstein, "Temperature and Charge Transfer in Re-ceptor Membrane," *Science* 132 (1960):841.

81. Robert Becker and G. Selden, *The Body Electric: Electromagnetism and the Foundation of Life* (New York: William Morrow and Co., 1985).

82. Ibid.

83. Ibid.

84. F. A. Brown, "Persistent Activity Rhythms in the Oyster," *Am. J. Physiology* 178 (1954):510.

85. Georges Lakhovsky, *The Secret of Life* (Whitefish, Mont.: Kessinger Pub. Co., 1939).

86. Becker and Selden.

87. Becker and Selden.

88. Becker and Selden.

89. Becker and Selden.

90. William Reich, *The Bioelectric Investigation of Sexuality and Anxiety* (New York: Farrar, Straus & Giroux, 1982).

91. Ibid.

92. Ibid.

93. Ibid.

94. Ibid.

95. Ibid.

96. Wilhelm Reich, *The Discovery of the Orgone* (New York: Noonday Press, 1942).

97. *Newsweek*, May 29, 1995, p. 69.

98. Harold Saxton Burr, *Blueprint for Immortality: The Electric Patterns of Light* (Essex, United Kingdom: C.W. Daniels Co., 1972).

99. Ibid.

100. C. W. Leadbeater, *The Chakras* (Wheaton, Ill.: Theosophical Publishing House, 1927).

101. Ibid.

102. Irvin Korr, Collected papers of Irvin M. Korr, American Academy of Osteopathy, Indianapolis, 1997.

103. Antonio Damasio, *Looking for Spinoza: Joy, Sorrow, and the Feeling Brain* (Orlando, FL: Harcourt Pub., 2003).

104. M. I. Bierenbaum, *Lancet*, May 3,1975, 1008–10.

105. *New England Journal of Medicine*, 1994, 330.2, 96-99; *Fluoride*, 1007, 30.2, 89–104.

106. *Calcif. Tissue Research*, 1974, 10:283–289.

107. F. Batmanghelidj, *Your Body's Many Cries for Water* (Falls Church, Va.: Global Health Solutions, P. O. Box 3189, 1992).

108. Bureau of Geology and Mines, Rolla, Missouri, *Classification of Mineral Waters at Excelsior Springs*, Missouri, 1919.

109. Hippocrates, trans. W. H. S. Jones (London: William Heinemann, 1931), 129, 1125.

110. Francis Adams, ed., *The Genuine Works of Hippocrates* (New York: William Wood & Co., 1929), 156–57.

111. Collection of Clarence W. Hansell, State University of New York, Stony Brook, NY, 1970.

112. Y. T. Shinobara and S. A. Tasber, "Successful Use of Boric Acid to Control Azole-Refractory Candida Vaginitis in a Woman with AIDS," *J. Acquired Immune Deficiency Syndrome and Human Retrovirology* 97, no. 16(3) (1997):219–20.

BIBLIOGRAPHY

Adams, Francis, ed. *The Genuine Works of Hippocrates.* New York: William Wood & Co, 1929.

Aeschbach, D., L. Sher, T. T. Postolache, J. R. Matthews, M. A. Jackson, and T. A. Wehr. "A Longer Biological Night in Long Sleepers than in Short Sleepers." *J. Clin. Endocrinol. Metab.* 88, no. 1 (2003):26–30.

Ajwani, S., K. J. Mattila, T. O. Narhi, R. S. Tilvis, and A. Ainamo. "Oral Health Status, C-Reactive Protein and Mortality—A 10-Year Follow-up Study." *Gerontology* 20, no. 1 (2003):32–40.

Anderson, R. E., T. A. Wadden, S. J. Bartlett, B. Zemel, T. J. Verde, and S. C. Franckowiak. "Effects of Lifestyle Activity vs. Structured Aerobic Exercise in Obese Women: A Randomized Trial." *JAMA* 281, no. 4 (1999):335–40.

Andrews, L. B. et al. "An Alternative Strategy for Studying Adverse Events in Medical Care." *Lancet* 349 (1997):309–13.

Antell, D. E., and E. M. Taczanowski. "How Environment and Lifestyle Choices Influence the Aging Process." *Ann. Plast. Surg.* 43, no. 6 (Dec. 1999):585–88.

Aparasu, R. R. "Visits to Office-Based Physicians in the United States for Medication-Related Morbidity." *J. Am. Pharm. Assoc.* 39 (1999):332–37.

Aparasu, R. R., and S. E. Fliginger. "Inappropriate Medication Prescribing for the Elderly by Office-Based Physicians." *Ann. Pharmacother.* 31 (1997):823–29.

Appleton, R. *The Catholic Encyclopedia: Holy Water.* Appleton, N.Y.: Encyclopedia Press, 1907.

Arnulf, I., P. Quintin, J. C. Alvarez, L. Vigil, Y. Touitou, A. L Lebre, A. Bellenger, O. Varoquaux, J. P. Derenne, J. F. Allilaire, C. Benkelfat, and

M. Leboyer. "Mid-Morning Tryptophan Depletion Delays REM Sleep Onset in Healthy Subjects." *Neuropsychopharmacology* 27, no. 5 (2002):843–51.

Atkins, R. C. *Dr. Atkins' New Diet Revolution* (New York: HarperCollins, 2002).

Bank, A. J. et al. "Relation of C-Reactive Protein and Other Cardiovascular Risk Factors to Penile Vascular Disease in Men with Erectile Dysfunction." *Int. J. Impot. Res.* 15, no. 4 (2003):231–36.

Barretti, P., and V.A. Soared. "Acute Renal Failure: Clinical Outcome and Causes of Death." *Ren. Fail.* 19 (1997):253–57.

Batmanghelidj, F. *Your Body's Many Cries for Water.* Falls Church, Va.: Global Health Solutions, P. O. Box 3189, 1992.

Becker, R. O., and G. Selden. *The Body Electric: Electromagnetism and the Foundation of Life.* New York: William Morrow and Co, 1985.

Bedell, S. E. "Incidence and Characteristics of Preventable Iatrogenic Cardiac Arrests." *JAMA* 265 (1991):2815–20.

Beinfield, H., and E. Korngold. *Between Heaven and Earth.* New York: Ballantine, 1991.

Ben-Eliyahu, S. "The Promotion of Tumor Metastasis by Surgery and Stress: Immunological Basis and Implications for Psychoneuroimmunology." *Brain Behav. Immun.* 1 (2003):527–36.

Bennett, R. M. "Adult Growth Hormone Deficiency in Patients with Fibromyalgia." *Curr. Rheumatol. Rep.* 4, no. 4 (2002):306–12.

Berton, E., D. Hoover, H. Fein, R. Galloway, and R. Smallridge. "Adaptation to Chronic Stress in Military Trainees: Adrenal Androgens, Testosterone, Glucocorticoids, IGF-1 and Immune Function. Dehydroepiandrosterone (DHEA) and Aging." New York: New York Academy of Sciences Meeting, June 17–19, 1995.

Berwick, D. M., and L. L. Leape. "Reducing Errors in Medicine." *British Med. J.* 319 (1999):136–37.

Black, P. H. "The Inflammatory Response is an Integral Part of the Stress Response: Implications for Atherosclerosis, Insulin Resistance, Type II Diabetes and Metabolic Syndrome X." *Brain Behav. Immun.* 17, no. 5 (2003):350–64.

Blair, S. N., Y. Cheng, and J. S. Holder. "Is Physical Activity or Physical Fitness More Important in Defining Health Benefits?" *Med. Sci. Sports Exerc.* 33, no. 6 Suppl. (June 2001):S379–99.

Bonghan, Kim. "Current Trends and Relations of the Meridian System." Pyongyang School of Medicine, Taegu, Korea, August 1961.

Brown, F. A. "Persistent Activity Rhythms in the Oyster." *Am. J. Physiol.* 178 (1954):510.

Bureau of Geology and Mines, Rolla, Missouri. *Classification of Mineral Waters at Excelsior Springs, Missouri,* 1919.

Burr, Harold Saxton. *Blueprint for Immortality: The Electric Patterns of Light.* Essex, United Kingdom:C.W. Daniels Co., 1972.

Butt, D. S. "The Sexual Response as Exercise: A Brief Review and Theoretical Proposal." *Sports Med.* 9, no. 6 (June 1990):330–43.

Cajochen, C., K. Krauchi, and A. Wirz-Justice. "Role of Melatonin in the Regulation of Human Circadian Rhythms and Sleep." *J. Neuroendocrinol.* 15, no. 4 (2003):432–37.

Callaghan, B. D. "Does the Pineal Gland Have a Role in the Psychological Mechanisms Involved in the Progression of Cancer?" *Med. Hypothesis* 59, no. 3 (2002):302–11.

Cannon, W. B. *The Wisdom of the Body.* New York: Norton, 1939.

Cappola, A. R., Q. L. Xue, L. Ferfucci, J. M. Guralnik, S. Volpato, and L. P. Fried. "Insulin-like Growth Factor I and Interleukin-6 Contribute Synergistically to Disability and Mortality in Older Women." *J. Clin. Endocrinol. Metab.* 88, no. 5(2003):2019–25.

Cardinali, D. P., M. G. Ladizesky, V. Boggio, R. A. Cutrera, and C. Mautalen. "Melatonin Effects on Bone: Experimental Facts and Clinical Perspectives." *J. Pineal Res.* 34, no. 2 (2003):81–87.

Carter, J. B., E. W. Banister, and A. P. Blaber. "Effect of Endurance Exercise on Autonomic Control of Heart Rate." *Sports Med.* 33, no. 1 (2003):33–46.

Casas, M., S. Ferre, and J. Rodriguez. "Methylxanthines Cause a Decrease of Prolactin Plasma Levels in Healthy Non-pregnant Women." *Human Neuropharmacology* 4 (1989):33–39.

Cerutti, E. *Mystic with the Healing Hands.* New York: Harper and Row, 1975.

Chen, J., J. He, L. Hamm, V. Batuman, and P. K. Whelton. "Serum Antioxidant Vitamins and Blood Pressure in the United States Population." *Hypertension* 40 (2002):810.

Cheng, X. *Chinese Acupuncture and Moxibustion.* Beijing: Foreign Language Press, 1987.

Chernen, L., S. Friedman, N. Goldberg, A. Feit, T. Kwan, and R. Stein. "Cardiac Disease and Nonorganic Chest Pain: Factors Leading to Disability." *Cardiology* 86, no. 1 (1995):15–21.

Clarkson-Smith, L., and A. A. Hartley. "Relationships Between Physical Exercise and Cognitive Abilities in Older Adults." *Psychology and Aging* 4, no. 2 (1989):183–89.

Cleare, A. J. "The Neuroendocrinology of Chronic Fatigue Syndrome." *Endocr. Rev.* 24, no. 2 (2003):236–52.

Coleridge, J., et al. "Survey of Drug-Related Deaths in Victoria." *Med. J. Austr.* 157 (1992):459–62.

Cooper, J. W. "Adverse Drug Reaction-Related Hospitalizations of Nursing Facility Patients: A 4-Year Study." *So. Med. J.* 92 (1999):485–90.

Cooper, Kenneth. *Aerobics.* New York: Bantam, 1973.

———. *The New Aerobics.* New York: Bantam, 1977.

———. *The Aerobics Way.* New York: Bantam, 1981.

Damasio, Antonio. *Looking for Spinoza: Joy, Sorrow, and the Feeling Brain.* Orlando, Fla.: Harcourt Pub. Co., 2003.

Davidson, W., D. W. Molloy, and M. Bedard. "Physician Characteristics and Prescribing for Elderly People in New Brunswick: Relation to Patient Outcomes." *CMAJ* 152(1995):1227–34.

Deadman, P., and M. Al-Khafaji. *A Manual of Acupuncture.* East Sussex, England: *Journal of Chinese Medicine Publication,* 1998.

DeVries, H. A., and G. M. Adams. "Electromyographic Comparison of Single Doses of Exercise and Meprobamate as to Effects on Muscular Relaxation." *Am. J. Phys. Med.* 51, no. 3 (1972):130–41.

DeVries, H. A., R. A. Wiswell, R. Bulbulian, and T. Moritani. "Tranquilizer Effect of Exercise." *Am. J. Phys. Med.* 60, no. 2 (1981):57–66.

Dik, M. G., S. M. Pluijm, C. Jonker, D. J. Deeg, M. Z. Lomecky, and P. Lips. "Insulin-like Growth Factor (IGF-1) and Cognitive Decline in Older Persons." *Neurobiol. Aging* 24, no. 2 (2003): 573–81.

Donchin, Y. et al. "A Look into the Nature and Causes of Human Errors in the Intensive Care Unit." *Crit. Care Med.* 23 (1995):294–300.

Drewnowski, A., and W. J. Evana. "Nutrition, Physical Activity, and Quality of Life in Older Adults: Summary." *J. Gerontol. A. Biol. Sci. Med. Sci.* 56, Spec. No. 2 (Oct 2001):89–94.

Duncan, J. J., J. E. Farr, J. Upton, R. D. Hagan, M. E. Oglesby, and S. N. Blair. "The Effects of Aerobic Exercise on Plasma Catecholamines and Blood Pressure in Patients with Mild Essential Hypertension." *JAMA* 254, no. 18 (1985):2609–13.

Dunn, A. L., B. H. Marcus, J. B. Kampert, M. E. Garcia, H. W. Kohl, and S. N. Blair. "Comparison of Lifestyle and Structured Interventions to Increase Physical Activity and Cardiorespiratory Fitness: A Randomized Trial." *JAMA* 281, no. 4 (1999):327–34.

Durlach, J., N. Pages, P. Bac, M. Bara, and A. Guiet-Bara. "Biorhythms and Possible Central Regulation of Magnesium Status, Phototherapy, Darkness Therapy and Chronopathological Forms of Magnesium Depletion." *J. Magnes. Res.* 15, no. 1–2 (2002):49–66.

Eichner, E. R. "The Hematology of Inactivity." *Rheum. Dis. Clin. North Am.* 16, no. 4 (Nov. 1990):815–25.

Ellis, A., N. Wiseman, and K. Boss. *Fundamentals of Chinese Acupuncture.* Brookline, Mass.: Paradigm Publications, 1988.

Everson, S. A. et al. "Hopelessness and 4-Year Progression of Carotid Atherosclerosis: The Kuopio Ischemic Heart Disease Risk Factor Study." *Arteriosclerosis, Thrombosis and Vascular Biol.* 17, no. 8 (1997):1490–95.

Eysenck, H. J. "Personality, Stress and Cancer: Prediction and Prophylaxis." *British J. of Med. Psychology* 61 (1988):57–75.

Figueroa, A., S. B. Going, L. A. Milliken, R. Blew, S. Sharp, and T. G. Lohman. "Body Composition Modulates the Effects of Hormone Replacement Therapy on Growth Hormone and Insulin-like Growth Factor-I Levels in Postmenopausal Women." *Gynecol. Obstet. Invest.* 54, no. 4 (2002):201–6.

Ford, E. S. "C-Reactive Protein Concentration and Cardiovascular Disease Risk Factors in Children: Findings from the National Health and Nutrition Examination Survey 1999–2000." *Circulation* 108, no. 9 (2003):1157–63.

Ford, E. S., S. Liu, D. M. Mannino, W. H. Giles, and S. J. Smith. "C-Reactive Protein Concentration and Concentrations of Blood Vitamins, Carotenoids, and Selenium among United States Adults." *Eur. J. Clin. Nutr.* 57, no. 9 (2003):1053–58.

Franks, Felix, ed. *Water: A Comprehensive Treatise.* Vol. 1. New York: Plenum Press, 1972.

Gandhi, T. K. "Drug Complications in Outpatients." *J. Gen. and Int. Med.* 15 (2000):149–54.

Garg, A. N., V. Singh, R. G. Weginwar, and V. N. Sagdeo. "An Elemental Correlation Study in Cancerous and Normal Breast Tissue with Successive Clinical Stages by Neutron Activation Analysis." *Biol. Trace Elem. Res.* 46, no. 3 (1994):185–202.

Gavrilov, L. A. and N. S. Gavrilov. "Season of Birth and Human Longevity." *J. of Anti-Aging Medicine* 2 (1999):365–66.

Gillberg, M. "Sleepiness and its Relation to the Length, Content, and Continuity of Sleep." *J. Sleep Res.* 4, no. 2 (1995):37–40.

Gillum, R. "Distribution of Serum Total Homocysteine and Its Association with Diabetes and Cardiovascular Risk Factors of the Insulin Resistance Syndrome in Mexican-American Men: The Third National Health and Nutrition Examination Survey." *Nutrition Journal* 2 (2003):6–21.

Gleick, J. *Faster: The Acceleration of Just About Everything.* New York: Pantheon, 1999.

Godfrey, R. J., Z. Madgwick, and G. P. Whyte. "The Exercise-Induced Growth Hormone Response in Athletes." *Sports Med.* 33, no. 8 (2003):599–613.

Gosney, M., and R. Tallis. "Prescription of Contraindicated and Interacting Drugs in Elderly Patients Admitted to Hospital." *Lancet* 2 (1984):564–67.

Grady, D. "Study Links Bipolar Drug to Fewer Suicides." *New York Times.* Sept. 17, 2003.

Gray, S. L., J. E. Mahoney, and D. K. Blough. "Adverse Drug Events in Elderly Patients Receiving Home Health Services Following Hospital Discharge." *Ann. Pharmacother.* 33 (1999):1147–53.

Grey, Alex. *Sacred Mirrors.* Rochester, Vt.: Inner Traditions International, 1990.

Habra, M. E., W. Linden, J. C. Anderson, and J. Weinberg. "Type D Personality Is Related to Cardiovascular and Neuroendocrine Reactivity to Acute Stress." *J. Psychosom. Res.* 55, no. 3 (2003):235–45.

Hambrecht, R., A. Wolf, S. Gielen, A. Linke, J. Hofer, S. Erbs, N. Schoene, and G. Schuler. "Effect of Exercise on Coronary Endothelial Function in Patients with Coronary Artery Disease." *NEJM* 342, no. 7 (2000):454–59.

Hammer, L. *Dragon Rises, Red Bird Flies.* New York: Barrytown/Station Hill, 1990.

Hansell, Clarence. Collection of State University of N.Y., Stony Brook, N.Y., 1970.

Helms, J. M. *Acupuncture Energetics: A Clinical Approach for Physicians.* Berkeley, Calif.: Medical Acupuncture Publishers, 1995.

Hermesh, H., A. Shalev, and H. Munitz. "Contributions of Adverse Drug Reaction to Admission in an Acute Psychiatric Ward." *ACTA Psychiat. Scan.* 72 (1985):104–10.

Hicks, R. A., and D. Picchioni. "Fluctuations in Sleep Duration Are Correlated with Salience of Stressful Experience." *Percept. Motor Skills* 96, no. 3, Pt. 2 (2003):1139–40.

Higashi, Y., S. Sasaki, K. Nakagawa, M. Kimura, K. Noma, S. Sasaki, K. Hara, H. Matsuura, C. Goto, T. Oshima, K. Chayama, and M. Yoshizumi. "Low Body Mass Index Is a Risk Factor for Impaired Endothelium-Dependent Vasodilation in Humans: Role of Nitric Oxide and Oxidative Stress." *J. Am. Coll. Cardiol.* 42, no. 2 (2003):256–63.

Hippocrates, W. H. S. Jones, trans. London: William Heinemann, 1931.

Hiura, M., T. Kikuchi, K. Nagasaki, and M. Uchiyama. "Elevation of Serum C-Reactive Protein Levels is Associated with Obesity in Boys." *Hypertens. Res.* 26, no. 7 (2002):541–46.

Holloszy, J. O. "Muscle Metabolism During Exercise." *Arch. Phys. Med. Rehabil.* 63 (1982):231–34.

Horne, J., and A.J. Reid. "Nighttime Sleep EEG Changes Following Body Heating in a Warm Bath." *Electroencephalography and Clin. Neurophysiology* 60 (1985):154–57. http://www.drunvalo.net/livingwater.html.

Ishiko, N., and W. R. Lowenstein. "Temperature and Charge Transfer in Receptor Membrane." *Science* 132 (1960):1841.

Jonasson, B., U. Jonasson, and T. Saldeen. "The Manner of Death Among Fatalities Where Dextropropoxyphene Caused or Contributed to Death." *Forensic. Sci. Int.* 96 (1998):181–87.

Jonasson, L., A. Wikby, and A. G. Olsson. "Low Serum Beta-Carotene Reflects Immune Activation in Patients with Coronary Artery Disease." *Nutr. Metab. Cardiovasc. Dis.* 13, no. 3 (2003):120–25.

Jorup-Ronstrom, C. A. "Prospective Study on the Amount, Spectrum, and Cost of Medical Disturbances in a Department of Infectious Diseases." *Scan. J. Infect. Dis. Suppl.* 36 (1982):150–56.

Justice, B. *Who Gets Sick*. New York: St. Martins, 1988.

Kahana, E., R. H. Lawrence, B. Kahana, K. Kercher, A. Wisniewski, E. Stoller, J. Tobin, and K. Stange. "Long-Term Impact of Preventive Proactivity on Quality of Life of the Old-Old." *Psychosom. Med.* 64, no. 3 (May–June 2002):382–94.

Kahleova, R., D. Palyzova, K. Zvara, J. Zvarova, K. Hrach, I. Novakova, J. Hyanek, B. Bendlova, and V. Kozich. "Essential Hypertension in Adolescents: Association with Insulin Resistance and with Metabolism of Homocysteine and Vitamins." *Am. J. Hypertens.* 15, no. 10, Pt. 1 (2002):857–64.

Kaptchuk, T. *Chinese Medicine: The Web That Has No Weaver.* New York: McGraw-Hill, 2000.

Kempner, Walter. "Compensation of Renal Metabolic Dysfunction: Treatment of Kidney Disease and Hypertensive Vascular Disease with the Rice Diet, III." *North Carolina Med. J.* 6 (1945):131–41.

Khalsa, D. S. "Integrated Medicine and the Prevention and Reversal of Memory Loss." *Altern. Ther. Health Med.* 4, no. 6 (Nov. 1998):38–43.

Kiecolt-Glaser, J. K., L. McGuire, T. F. Robles, and R. Glaser. "Emotions, Morbidity, and Mortality: New Perspectives from Psychoneuroimmunology." *Annual Rev. Psychol.* 53 (2002):83–107.

Kiecolt-Glaser, J. K., L. McGuire, T. F. Robles, and R. Glaser. "Psychoneuroimmunology: Psychological Influences on Immune Function and Health." *J. Consult. Clin. Psychol.* 70, no. 3 (2002):537–47.

Kiecolt-Glaser, J. K., L. McGuire, T. F. Robles, and R. Glaser. "Psychoneuroimmunology and Psychosomatic Medicine: Back to the Future." *Psychosom. Med.* 64, no. 1 (2002):15–28.

Kimball, H. R., and R. G. Petersdorf. "Back to the Future for Internal Medicine." *Am. J. Med.* 104 (1998):315–16.

Kirsch, I., and T. J. Moore. "The Emperor's New Drugs: An Analysis of Antidepressant Medication Data Submitted to the U.S. Food and Drug Administration." *Prevention and Treatment* 5 (July 15, 2002):Article 23.

Knowles, J. *The Responsibility of the Individual.* Cambridge, Mass.: *Journal of the American Academy of Arts and Sciences,* 1977.

Kolata, G. "Research Suggests More Health Care May Not Be Better." *New York Times.* July 21, 2002.

Korr, Irvin. Collected papers of Irvin M. Korr, American Academy of Osteopathy, Indianapolis, 1997.

Kozielcec, T., B. Starobrat-Hermelin, and L. Kotkowiak. "Deficiency of Certain Trace Elements in Children Leads to Hyperactivity." *Psychiatry Pol.* 28, no. 3 (1994):345–53.

Krachler, M., M. Lindschinger, B. Eber, N. Watzinger, and S. Wallner. "Trace Elements in Coronary Heart Disease: Impact of Intensified Lifestyle and Modification from Biological Trace Elements." *Biol. Trace Elem. Res.* 60 (1997):175–85.

Krauchi, K., C. Cajochen, E. Werth, and A. Wirz-Justice. "Alteration of Internal Circadian Phase Relationships after Morning versus Evening Carbohydrate-Rich Meals in Humans." *J. Biol. Rhythms* 17, no. 4 (2002):364–76.

Kraus, H., W. Nagler, and S. Weber. "Role of Exercise in the Prevention of Disease." *GP* 20, no. 3 (1959):121–26.

Kraus, H., and S. Weber. "Back Pain and Tension Syndromes in a Sedentary Profession." *Arch. Env. Health* 4 (1962):38–44.

Krizkova, L., Z. Durackova, J. Sandula, D. Slamenova, and V. Sasinkova. "Fungal Beta-1-3-D-Glucan Derivatives Exhibit High Antioxidative and Antimutagenic Activity in Vitro." *Anticancer Res.* 23, no. 3B (2003):2751–56.

Lakhovsky, Georges. *The Secret of Life*. Whitefish, Mont.: Kessinger Pub. Co., 1939.

LaVert, M. S., M. Moore-Ede, and S. Campbell. *The Complete Idiot's Guide to Getting a Good Night's Sleep*. New York: Alpha Books, 1998.

Lazarou, J., B. H. Pomeranz, and P. N. Corey. "Incidence of Adverse Drug Reactions in Hospitalized Patients: A Meta-Analysis of Prospective Studies." *JAMA* 279 (1998):1200–05.

Leadbeater, C. W. *The Chakras*. Wheaton, Ill.: Theosophical Publishing House, 1927.

Lee, I. M., C. C. Hsieh, and R. S. Paffenbarger, Jr. "Exercise Intensity and Longevity in Men: The Harvard Alumni Health Study." *JAMA* 273, no. 15 (Apr. 19, 1995):1179–84.

Lee, I. M., R. S. Paffenbarger, Jr., and C. H. Hennekens. "Physical Activity, Physical Fitness, and Longevity." *Aging (Milano)* 9, no. 1–2 (April 1997):2–11.

Lee, I. M. and R. S. Paffenbarger, Jr. "Associations of Light, Moderate, and Vigorous Intensity Physical Activity with Longevity: The Harvard Alumni Study." *Am. J. Epidemiol.* 151, no. 3 (Feb. 1, 2000):293–99.

Lefevre, F. et al. "Iatrogenic Complications in High-Risk, Elderly Patients." *Arch. Intern. Med.* 153 (1992):2074–80.

Leskowitz, E. D. "Is Depression a Risk Factor for Ischemic Stroke?" *Complementary and Alternative Med.* 3, no. 2 (2002):1–2.

Levy, M. et al. "Computerized Surveillance of Adverse Drug Reactions in Hospital Implementation." *Eur. J. Clin. Pharmacol.* 104 (1998):887–92.

Lim, U., and P. A. Cassano. "Homocysteine and Blood Pressure in the Third National Health and Nutrition Examination Survey, 1988–1994." *Am. J. Epidemiol.* 156, no. 12 (2002):1105–13.

Lindley, C. M. "Inappropriate Medication Is a Major Cause of Adverse Drug Reactions in Elderly Patients." *Age and Ageing* 4 (1992):294–300.

Lowe, G. et al. "Total Tooth Loss and Prevalent Cardiovascular Disease in Men and Women: Possible Roles of Citrus Fruit Consumption, Vitamin C, and Inflammatory and Thrombotic Variables." *J. Clin. Epidemiol.* 56, no. 7 (2003):694–700.

Luboshitzky, R., U. Ophir, R. Nave, R. Epstein, Z. Shen-Orr, and P. Herer. "The Effect of Pyridoxine Administration on Melatonin Secretion in Normal Men." *Neuroendocrinol. Lett.* 23, no. 3 (2002):213–17.

Malik, I. A., P. Foy, M. Wallymahmed, J. P. Wilding, and I. A. MacFarlane. "Assessment of Quality of Life in Adults Receiving Long-Term Growth Hormone Replacement Compared to Control Subjects." *Clin. Endocrinol.* 59, no. 1 (2003):75–81.

Manetta, J., J. F. Brun, C. Fedou, L. Maimom, C. Prefaut, and J. Mercier. "Serum Levels of Insulin-like Growth Factor (IFG-1) and IGF-Protein Binding Proteins-1 and -3 in Middle-Aged and Young Athletes vs. Sedentary Men: Relationship with Glucose Disposal." *Metabolism* 52, no. 7 (2003):821–26.

Mann, F. *The Treatment of Disease by Acupuncture.* 2d ed. London: William Heinemann Medical Books Ltd., 1971.

———. *Scientific Aspects of Acupuncture.* London: William Heinemann Medical Books, 1977.

Martin, R. M. et al. "Underreporting of Suspected Adverse Drug Reactions to Newly Marketed ("Black Triangle") Drugs in General Practice: Observational Study." *British Med. J.* 317 (1998):119–20.

Maruta, T., R. C. Colligan, M. Malinchoc, and K. P. Offord. "Optimists vs. Pessimists: Survival Rate among Medical Patients over a 30-Year Period." *Mayo Clin. Proc.* 75 (2000):140–43.

Mayer, J., P. Roy, and K. P. Mitra. "Relation Between Caloric Intake, Body Weight, and Physical Work: Studies in an Industrial Male Population in West Bengal." *Am. J. Clin. Nutr.* 4, no. 2 (1956):169–75.

McDonald, S. P., G. P. Maguire, N. Duarte, X. L. Wang, and W. E. Hoy. "C-Reactive Protein, Cardiovascular Risk, and Renal Disease in a Remote Australian Aboriginal Community." *Clin. Sci. (London)* E-pub ahead of print (2003).

McKeown, T. *The Role of Medicine: Dream, Mirage, or Nemesis.* Princeton, N.J.: Princeton University Press, 1979.

Melchizedek, Drunvalo. *Water, The Source of Life.* Santa Fe: Clear Light, 1999.

Mendosa, R. *The Glycemic Index.* New York: Avery Press, 2001.

Merrill, M. M., J. C. Miller, J. J. Lipsitz, J. K. Walsh, and C. D. Wylie. "The Sleep of Long-Haul Truck Drivers." *NEJM* 337, no. 11 (1997):755–61.

Mitchell, A. A. et al. "Drug Utilization and Reported Adverse Reactions in Hospitalized Children." *Am. J. Epidemiol.* 110 (1979):196–204.

Moore-Ede, M. *The Twenty-four Hour Society.* New York: Addison-Wesley, 1993.

Myers, J., M. Prakash, V. Froelicher, S. Partington, and J. E. Atwood. "Exercise Capacity and Mortality among Men Referred for Exercise Testing." *NEJM* 346, no. 11 (2002):793–801.

Natale, V., A. Adan, and J. Chotai. "Further Results on the Association Between Morningness-Eveningness Preference and the Season of Birth in Human Adults." *Neuropsychobiology* 46 (2002):209–14.

National Center for Health Statistics. *Health: United States, 1993.* Hyattsville, Md.: Public Health Service, 1994.

Nelson, C. J., B. Rosenfeld, W. Breitbart, and M. Galietta. "Spirituality, Religion, and Depression in the Terminally Ill." *Psychosomatics* 43, no. 3 (2002):213–20.

Nelson, K. M., and R. L. Talbert. "Drug-Related Hospital Admissions." *Pharmacotherapy* 16 (1996):701–07.

Newsweek, May 29, 1995, p. 69.

New York Times. "Investigators Find Repeated Deception in Ads for Drugs." December 4, 2002; "Doctors Are Reminded, 'Wash Up!'" November 9, 1999.

Nias, D. K. "Therapeutic Effects of Low-Level Direct Electrical Currents." *Psychol. Bull.* 83(1976):766.

Norman, A., R. Bellocco, A. Bergstrom, and A. Wolk. "Validity and Reproducibility of Self-Reported Total Physical Activity—Differences by Relative Weight." *Int. J. Obes. Relat. Metab. Disord.* 25, no. 5 (May 2001):682–88.

Orr, L. *Breaking the Death Habit: The Science of Everlasting Life.* Berkeley, Calif.: Frog Ltd., 1998.

Ottervanger, J. P. et al. "Differences in Perceived and Presented Adverse Drug Reactions in General Practice." *J. Clin. Epidemiol.* 51 (1998):795–99.

Paffenbarger, R. S., Jr., R. T. Hyde, A. L. Wing, and C. C. Hsieh. "Physical Activity, All-Cause Mortality, and Longevity of College Alumni." *NEJM* 314, no. 10 (March 6, 1986):605–13.

Paffenbarger, R. S., Jr., R. T. Hyde, A. L. Wing, I. M. Lee, D. L. Jung, and J. B. Kampert. "The Association of Changes in Physical Activity Level and Other Lifestyle Characteristics with Mortality Among Men." *NEJM* 328, no. 8 (Feb. 25, 1993):538–45.

Paffenbarger, R. S., Jr., S. N. Blair, and I. M. Lee. "A History of Physical Activity, Cardiovascular Health, and Longevity: The Scientific Contributions of Jeremy N. Morris, DSc, DPH, FRCP." *Int. J. Epidemiol.* 30, no. 5 (Oct. 2001):1184–92.

Page, J. and D. Henry. "Consumption of NSAIDs and the Development of Congestive Heart Failure in Elderly Patients: An Underrecognized Public Health Problem." *Arch. Int. Med.* 1601 (2000):777–84.

Palmblad, J., B. Petrini, J. Wassereman, and T. Akerstedt. "Lymphocyte and Granulocyte Reactions During Sleep Deprivation." *Psychosomatic Med.* 41, no. 4 (1979):273–80.

Pawlikowski, M., M. Kolomecka, A. Wojtczak, and M. Karasek. "Effects of Six Months Melatonin Treatment on Sleep Quality and Serum Concentrations of Estradiol, Cortisol, Dehydroepiandrosterone Sulfate, and Somatomedin C in Elderly Women." *Neuroendocrinol. Lett.* 23, no. Suppl. 1 (2002):17–19.

Payette, H., R. Roubenoff, P. F. Jacques, C. A. Dinarello, P. W. Wilson, L. W. Abad, and T. Harris. "Insulin-like Growth Factor-1 and Interleukin 6 Predict Sarcopenia in Very Old Community-Living Men and Women: The Framingham Heart Study." *Am. Geriatr. Soc.* 51, no. 9 (2003):1237–43.

Pelletier, K. *Longevity: Fulfilling Our Biological Potential.* New York: Delacorte, 1991.

Penninx, B. W. et al. "Inflammatory Markers and Depressed Mood in Older Persons: Results from the Health, Aging and Body Composition Study." *Biol. Psychiatry* 54, no. 5 (2003):566–72.

Physicians' Desk Reference. Montvale, N.J.: Medical Economics Co., 2001.

Raschke, R.A. et al. "A Computer Alert System to Prevent Injury from Adverse Drug Events: Development and Evaluation in a Community Teaching Hospital." *JAMA* 280 (1998):1317–20.

Reich, Wilhelm. *The Discovery of the Orgone.* New York: Noonday Press, 1942.

———. *The Bioelectric Investigation of Sexuality and Anxiety.* New York: Farrar, Straus, and Giroux, 1982.

Rein, Glen. "Biological Effects of Quantum Fields and Their Role in the Natural Healing Process." *Frontier Perspectives* 7(1998):16–23.

Renner, S. W., P. J. Howanitz, and P. Bachner. "Wristband Identification Error Reporting in 712 Hospitals: A College of American Pathologists' Q-Probes Study of Quality Issues in Transfusion Practice," *Arch. Path. Lab. Med.* 117 (1993):573–77.

Riemann, D., T. Klein, A. Rodenbeck, B. Feige, A. Horny, R. Hummel, G. Wesk, A. Al-Shajlawi, and U. Voderholzer. "Nocturnal Cortisol and Melatonin Secretion in Primary Insomnia." *Psychiatry Res.* 113, no. 1–2 (2002):17–27.

Ries, M. D., E. F. Philbin, and G. D. Groff. "Relationship Between Severity of Gonarthrosis and Cardiovascular Fitness." *Clin. Orthop.* 313 (April 1995):169–76.

Riolli, L., and V. Savicki. "Optimism and Coping as Moderators of the Relationship Between Chronic Stress and Burnout." *Psychol. Rep.* 92, no. 3, Pt. 2 (2003):1215–26.

Robin, Eugene D. *Matters of Life and Death: Risks vs. Benefits of Medical Care.* New York: W. H. Freeman & Co, 1984.

Rogers, R. L., J. S. Meyer, and K. F. Mortel. "After Reaching Retirement Age Physical Activity Sustains Cerebral Perfusion and Cognition." *J. Am. Geriatr. Soc.* 38 (1990):123–28.

Ross, C. E., and J. Moriwsky. "Family Relationships, Social Support, and Subjective Life Expectancy." *J. Health Soc. Behav.* 43, no. 4 (2002):469–89.

Rossouw, J. E. "Risks and Benefits of Estrogen Plus Progestin in Healthy Postmenopausal Women: Principal Results from the Women's Health Initiative Randomized Controlled Trial." *JAMA* 288 (2002):321–33.

Roth, G., M. Lane, D. Ingram, and S. Ball. "Studies Suggest Caloric Restriction in Monkeys May Extend Life." *J. Clin. Endocrin. and Metabolism* 82, no. 7 (1997):2093–96.

Ruiz-Torres, A., and M. Soares de Melo Kirzner. "Aging and Longevity are Related to Growth Hormone/Insulin-like Growth Factor-1 Secretion." *Gerontology* 48, no. 6 (2002):401–7.

Sandvik, L., J. Erikssen, E. Thaulow, E. Gunnar, R. Mundal, and K. Rodahl. "Physical Fitness as a Predictor of Mortality Among Healthy, Middle-Aged Norwegian Men." *NEJM* 328, no. 8 (1993):533–37.

Sankey, M. *Esoteric Acupuncture. Gateway to Expanded Healing.* Los Angeles: Mountain Castle Publishing, 1991.

Schnohr, P., J. Parner, and P. Lange. "Joggers Live Longer: The Osterbro Study." *Ugeskr. Laeger* 163, no. 19 (May 7, 2001):2633–35.

Selye, H. *The Physiology and Pathology of Exposure to Stress.* Montreal: ACTA, Inc., 1950.

Shealy, C. N., *DHEA: The Youth and Health Hormone.* Los Angeles: Keats, 1999.

Shealy, C. N., and C. M. Myss. *The Science of Medical Intuition.* Boulder, Colo.: Sounds True, 2002.

Shealy, C. N. *The Methuselah Potential for Health and Longevity*. Fair Grove, Mo.: Brindabella Books, 2002.

Shealy, C. N., T. Smith, S. Liss, and V. Borgmeyer. "EEG Alterations During Absent Healing." *Subtle Energies and Energy Medicine* 2, no. 3 (2002):241–248.

Sherman, S. E., R. B. D'Agostino, J. L. Cobb, and W. B. Kannel. "Does Exercise Reduce Mortality Rates in the Elderly? Experience from the Framingham Heart Study." *Am. Heart J.* 128, no. 5 (Nov. 1994):965–72.

Shi, Y. et al. "Stressed to Death: Implication of Lymphocyte Apoptosis for Psychoneuroimmunology." *Brain Behav. Immun.* 17, no. 1 (2003):S18–26.

Shinobara, Y. T., and S. A. Tasber. "Successful Use of Boric Acid to Control Azole-Refractory Candida Vaginitis in a Woman with AIDS." *J. Acquired Immune Deficiency Syndrome and Human Retrovirology* 97, no. 16(3)(1997): 219–20.

Sinoff, G., L. Ore, and D. Zlotogorsky. "Does the Presence of Anxiety Affect the Validity of a Screening Test for Depression in the Elderly?" *Int. J. Geriatr. Psychiatry* 17, no. 4 (2002):309–14.

Smith, C. "Permanent Changes in the Physico-chemical Properties of Water Following Exposure to Resonant Circuits." *J. Scientific Exploration* 15 (2001):5.

Spore, D. L. et al. "Inappropriate Drug Prescriptions for Elderly Residents of Board and Care Facilities." *Am. J. Pub. Health* 87 (1997):404–09.

Springfield News Leader. "Men's Flab Linked to Lack of Deep Sleep." Aug. 16, 2000, sec. B, p. 8.

Starfield, B. "Is U.S. Health Really the Best in the World?" *JAMA* 284, July 26 (2000): 483–85.

Stevens, J., J. Cai, K. R. Evenson, and R. Thomas. "Fitness and Fatness as Predictors of Mortality from All Causes and from Cardiovascular Disease in Men and Women in the Lippid Research Clinics Study." *Am. J. Epidemiol.* 156, no. 9 (Nov. 1, 2002):832–41.

Suzuki, K., R. Oyama, E. Hayashi, and Y. Arakawa. "Liver Diseases and Essential Trace Elements." *Nippon Rinsho* 54, no. 1 (1996):85–92.

Tafreshi, M. J. et al. "Medication-Related Visits to the Emergency Department: A Prospective Study." *Ann. Pharmacother.* 33 (1999):1252–57.

Takahashi, K. et al. "The Elevation of Natural Killer Cell Activity Induced by Laughter in a Crossover Designed Study." *Int. J. Mol. Med.* 8, no. 6 (2001):645–50.

Tecumseh, Chief, Shawnee Nation. Widely published on the Internet.

Thomas, C. B. "Observation of Some Precursors of Essential Hypertension and Coronary Artery Disease: Hypercholesterolemia in Healthy Young Adults." *Am. J. Am. Sciences* 232 (1956):391–96.

Thomas, C. B., K. R. Duszynski, and J. W. Shafer. "Family Attitudes Reported in Youth as Potential Predictors of Cancer." *Psychosomatic Med.* 41, no. 4 (1979):287–302.

Thomas, E. J., and T. A. Brennan. "Incidence and Types of Preventable Adverse Events in Elderly Patients: Population-Based Review of Medical Records." *British Med. J.* 310 (2000):741–44.

Thompson, Tommy. Speech delivered to American Medical Association, Chicago, Ill., July 18, 2002.

Thune, I., T. Brenn, E. Lund, and M. Gaard. "Physical Activity and the Risk of Breast Cancer." *NEJM* 336, no. 18 (1997):1269–75.

Tiller, William. Part of Acupuncture Symposium. Speech delivered to Stanford University, Acupuncture Symposium, Stanford University, Stanford, Calif., June 1972.

Tveramo, A., O. S. Dalgard, and B. Claussen. "Increasing Psychological Stress Among Young Adults in Norway, 1990–2000." *Tidsskr. Nor. Laegeforen* 123, no. 15 (2003):2011–15.

Unden, A. L., S. Elofsson, S. Knox, M. S. Lewitt, and K. Brismar. "IGF-I in a Normal Population: Relation to Psychosocial Factors." *Clin. Endocrinol.* 57, no. 6 (2002):793–803.

Vaillant, G. E. "The Association of Ancestral Longevity with Successful Aging." *J. Gerontol.* 46, no. 6 (Nov. 1991):P292–98.

Van Auken, J. *Edgar Cayce's Approach to Rejuvenation of the Body.* Virginia Beach, Va.: A.R.E. Press, 1996.

Vita, A. J., R. B. Perry, H. B. Hubert, and J. F. Fries. "Aging, Health Risks, and Cumulative Disability." *NEJM* 338, no. 15 (Apr. 9, 1998):1035–41.

Wang, B., L. Ma, and T. Liu. "406 Cases of Angina Pectoris in Coronary Heart Disease Treated with Saponin of Tribulus Terrestris." *Zhong Xi Yi Jie He Za Zhi* 10, no. 2 (1990):85–87.

Watson, G. *Nutrition and Your Mind: The Psychological Response.* New York: Bantam, 1978.

Weingart, S.N. et al. "Epidemiology of Medical Error." British Med. J. 310 (2000):774–77.

Worrall, A. *Essay on Prayer*. Fair Grove, Mo.: Self-Health Systems, 1982.

Yanchi, L. *The Essential Book of Traditional Chinese Medicine*. New York: Columbia University Press, 1988.

Zhu, B. T. "Hyperhomocysteinemia Is a Risk Factor for Estrogen-Induced Hormonal Cancer." *Int. J. of Oncology* 22 (2003):499–508.

Zisapel, N. "Melatonin-Dopamine Interactions: From Basic Neurochemistry to a Clinical Setting." *Cell Mol. Neurobiol.* 21, no. 6 (2001):605–16.

ADDITIONAL REFERENCES
OF INTEREST

1. H. Benson, *The Relaxation Response* (New York: William Morrow & Co., 1975).

2. *Biofeedback and Autogenic Training*, Biofeedback Certification Institute, 10200 West 44th Avenue, Suite 304, Wheat Ridge, CO 80033-2840, phone: (303)420-2902.

3. C. Bird, *The Life and Trials of Gaston Naessens* (St. Lambert, Quebec: Les Presses de l'Universate de la Persoune, Inc., 1990).

4. A. Cantwell, *The Cancer Miracle* (New York: Aries Rising Press, 1990).

5. R. H. Cox, C. N. Shealy, R. K. Cady, R. Cadle R, and G. Richards, "Successful Treatment of Rheumatoid Arthritis with GigaTENS™," *Journal of Neurological and Orthopaedic Medicine and Surgery* 17, no. 1 (1996):31.

6. M. Delhez, M. Hansenne, and J. J. Legros, "Testosterone and Depression in Men Aged over 50 Years. Andropause and psychopathology: Minimal Systemic Work-up," *Ann. Endocrinol. (Paris)* 64, no. 2 (2003):162–69.

7. W. B. Ershler and E. T. Keller, "Age-Associated Increased Interleukin-6 Gene Expression, Late-Life Diseases, and Frailty," *Annu. Rev. Med.* 51 (2000):245–70.

8. A. O. Fatusi et al., "Assessment of Andropause Awareness and Erectile Dysfunction among Married Men in Ile-Ife, Nigeria," *Aging Male* 7, no. 2 (2003):79–85.

9. J. Helms, *Acupuncture Energetics* (Medical Acupuncture Publishers, Berkeley, Calif., 1995).

10. S. W. Lamberts, A. W. Van den Beld, and A. J. Van der Lely, "The Endocrinology of Aging," *Science* 279(1998):305–06.

11. V. Livingston-Wheeler, *The Conquest of Cancer* (San Diego: Waterside Productions, 1984).

12. W. Luthe and J. H. Schultz, *Autogenic Therapy and Training* (a six-volume work) (Gruen and Stratton, New York, 1969).

13. U. Maier, "Hormone Profile in the Aging Man," *Wien. Med. Wochenschr.* 151, nos. 18–20 (2001):422–425.

14. H. Motoyama, *Theories of the Chakras: Bridge to Higher Consciousness* (Theosophical Publishing House, Wheaton, Ill., 1981).

15. S. N. Seidman, "Testosterone Deficiency and Mood in Aging Men: Pathogenic and Therapeutic Interactions," *World J. Biol. Psychiatry* 4, no. 1 (2003):14–20.

16. R. Shabsigh, L. Zakaria, A. G. Anastasiadis, and A. S. Seidman, "Sexual Dysfunction and Depression: Etiology, Prevalence, and Treatment," *Curr. Urol. Rep.* 6, no. 2 (2001):463–67.

17. C. N. Shealy, "A review of Dehydroepiandrosterone," *Integrated Physiological and Behavioral Science* 30, no. 4 (1995):308–313.

18. C. N. Shealy, *90 Days to Stress-Free Living* (Dorset, England: Element Books, 1993–1999).

19. C. N. Shealy, *Retraining the Nervous System—Biogenics® Program*. Cassette training tape.

20. C. N. Shealy, B. Borgmeyer, and P. Thomlinson, "Institution, Neurotensin and the Ring of Air," *Subtle Energies and Energy Medicine* 11, no. 2 (2002):145–50.

21. C. N. Shealy and C. M. Myss, "The Ring of Fire and DHEA: A Theory for Energetic Restoration of Adrenal Reserves," *Subtle Energies and Energy Medicine* 6, no. 2 (1995):167–75.

22. R. S. Tan and S. J. Pu, "Impact of Obesity on Hypogonadism in the Andropause," *Int. J. Androl.* 25, no. 4 (2002):195–201.

23. S. Vermeulen and J. M. Kaufman, "Aging of the Hypothalamo-Pituitary-Testicular Axis in Men," *Horm. Res.* 43, nos. 1–3 (1995):25–28.

INDEX

The letter f after a page number indicates an illustration.

Methuselah Promise, 192–93
Meuniere's Syndrome, 192
Micoid laminar crystals, 171, 172, 173
Microorganisms, 14–15
Microwaves, 123, 126
Migraines, 68, 143, 162, 187, 193–94
Mind, xv, 7, 138, 142, 154
Minerals, 144, 160
Minnesota Multiphasic Personality Inventory (MMPI), 99, 215
Mood, 125, 166, 170
Multiple sclerosis, 35, 86, 134, 194
Muscles, 68, 71, 128, 129, 141
    relaxation of, 61, 62–63
Music, 103, 104, 139, 154, 183, 184
Myss, Caroline, 2, 96, 153

Negative polarity, 215
Nerves, 150
    electricity and, 117, 118, 120
Nervous system, 49, 150
    autonomic, 6, 29, 68, 69
    central, 40, 54
    electromagnetic energy and, 121
    parasympathetic, 69, 70, 128, 129, 215
    sympathetic, 29, 69, 70, 90, 128, 129, 216
Neurochemicals, 136, 145, 187
Neurohormones, 91
Neurotensin, 37, 40–42, 124, 145, 187, 215
Neurotransmitter, 40
Norepinephrine (NE). See Adrenaline
Nursing homes, 11–12
Nutrition, 8, 9, 16, 60, 78–83, 89, 90, 137, 154, 183

Obesity, 19, 32, 33, 34, 70, 78, 83, 84, 156, 162, 194–95
    abdominal, 84
Obsessive-compulsive disorder, 195
Omega-3 fatty acids, 85, 189
Orgasm, 127–29, 145, 156
Orgone (life energy), 123, 147, 215
Ornithine, 34, 215
Osteopathy, 118, 119
Osteoporosis, 46–47, 51, 106, 160, 195
Out-of-body experience, 5
Ovulation, 107, 108
Oxidation, 31, 52
Oxidative stress, 51, 54
Ozone, 169
Ozone layer, 51

Pain, 167, 170
    chronic, 100, 101, 102, 138, 183
    relief of, 5, 40, 46, 47, 68, 143, 171
Pancreas, 29, 31, 126
Panic disorder, 35, 71, 179
Pasteur, Louis, 15
Pasteurization, 21
Past-life therapy, 5, 178
Periodontal disease, 106
Pharmaceutical industry, 14, 24–27
Pharmacology, 1
PharmacoMafia, 16, 24–27, 32
Phenylalanine, 35, 137, 215
Phobias, 71
Photostimulation, 66–67, 101–2, 104, 132, 139, 177, 184, 215
Physical anatomy, 115
Physical body, x–xvi, 7, 142, 152, 153
    electromagnetic energy and, 116, 122, 124–26, 131–40
    electromagnetic system of, xiii, 102, 116, 117, 118, 121, 122, 130
    energy field of, xiv, 148–50, 152, 214
Physical fitness, 70
Physical therapists, 68
Physics, 118, 123
Piezoelectricity, 102, 121, 122, 128, 129
Pineal gland, 142
Pituitary gland, 29, 40, 97, 106, 142, 153
Pneumonia, 23
Pollution, 54, 137
    electromagnetic, 137–38
Positive imagery, xiv
Positive polarity, 215
Positive thinking, 62
Potassium, 118, 120, 121, 128, 129, 187
Pregnenolone, 33, 215
Premenstrual syndrome (PMS), 141
Progesterone, 33, 57, 107, 110, 111, 112, 113, 215
    natural cream, 142, 185, 191, 192, 194, 197, 215
Progestrin, 17
Prostate, 110, 153
    disease/problems of, 108, 110, 195–96, 215
Psoriasis, 196
Psyche, xiii
Psychosis, 135, 167

Qi. See Chi
Quantum theory, 123
Quartz crystals, 102–4, 154, 172, 215

ABOUT THE AUTHOR

C. Norman Shealy, M.D., Ph.D., is a neurosurgeon, trained at Massachusetts General Hospital, after completing medical school at Duke University. He has taught at Harvard, Western Reserve, University of Wisconsin, University of Minnesota, and Forest Institute of Professional Psychology. He was the founding president of the American Holistic Medical Association. Currently he is the president of Holos University Graduate Seminary, which offers doctoral programs in Spiritual Healing and Energy Medicine. He introduced the concepts of Dorsal Column Stimulation and Transcutaneous Electrical Nerve Stimulation (TENS), both now used worldwide. In 1971 he founded the first comprehensive, holistic clinic for management of pain and stress management. The Shealy Institute became the most successful and most cost-effective pain clinic in the United States, with 85 percent success in more than 30,000 patients. The Shealy protocols for management of depression, migraine, fibromyalgia, and back pain are increasingly being integrated into hospitals and individual practices. The Shealy Wellness Center focuses now on these four major chronic problems.

Dr. Shealy holds nine patents for innovative discoveries, has published more than 300 articles and twenty-two books. His free e-newsletter is available at www.normshealy.net, and Holos University information can be found at www.hugs-edu.org.